PEDIATRICS CLERKSHIP

101 BIGGEST MISTAKES

AND HOW TO AVOID THEM

CLERKSHIP MISTAKE SERIES

PEDIATRICS CLERKSHIP

101 BIGGEST MISTAKES

AND HOW TO AVOID THEM

Andrew A. Bremer, M.D., Ph.D.
Bryan H. Goldstein, M.D.
Milton H. Nirken, M.D.
Samir P. Desai, M.D.

Foreword by Ralph D. Feigin, M.D.

PUBLISHED BY

MD2B

HOUSTON, TEXAS

www.MD2B.net

The Pediatrics Clerkship: 101 Biggest Mistakes and How to Avoid Them is published by MD2B, P.O. Box 300988, Houston, Texas 77230-0988.

NOTICE: The authors and publisher disclaim any personal liability, either directly or indirectly, for advice or information presented within. The authors and publisher have used care and diligence in the preparation of this book. Every effort has been made to ensure the accuracy and completeness of information contained within this book. The reader should understand, however, that most of the subject matter of the book is not rooted in scientific observation. The recommendations made within this book have come from the authors' personal experiences and interactions with other attending physicians, residents, and students over many years. Since expectations vary from medical school to medical school, clerkship to clerkship, and resident to resident, the recommendations are not universally applicable. No responsibility is assumed for errors, inaccuracies, omissions, or any false or misleading implication that may arise due to the text.

Printed in the United States of America

ISBN # 0-9725561-4-1

Contents

Part I: The Inpatient Environment

Chapter 1: Prerounds

Chapter 2: Work Rounds

Chapter 3: On Call

Chapter 4: Write-Ups

Chapter 5: The Oral Case Presentation

Chapter 6: The Daily Progress Note

Chapter 7: Attending Rounds

Part II: The Outpatient Environment

Chapter 8: Before Seeing the Patient (Outpatient Setting)

Chapter 9: While Seeing The Patient (Outpatient Setting)

Chapter 10: When Presenting the Patient
(Outpatient Setting)

Chapter 11: When Completing Clinic
Paperwork (Outpatient Setting)

Part III: The Nursery

Chapter 12: Prerounds (Nursery)

Chapter 13: Work Rounds (Nursery)

Chapter 14: On Call (Nursery)

Chapter 15: Write-Ups (Nursery)

Chapter 16: The Oral Case Presentation (Nursery)

Chapter 17: The Daily Progress Note (Nursery)

Chapter 18: Attending Rounds (Nursery)

About the Authors

Andrew A. Bremer, M.D., Ph.D.

Dr. Andrew Bremer obtained his B.S. degree in Molecular Biophysics and Biochemistry from Yale University in 1994, and received his M.D. degree *cum laude* and Ph.D. degree in Pharmacology from the Boston University School of Medicine in 2001. During medical school, he was elected into Alpha Omega Alpha, served as a lecturer in the Medical Pharmacology course, and received a student achievement award. He is currently a senior resident in the Combined Internal Medicine-Pediatrics Residency Program at the Baylor College of Medicine in Houston, Texas. During his residency, Dr. Bremer served as a Chief Internal Medicine-Pediatrics Resident and Chief Neonatology Resident.

In July 2005, Dr. Bremer will begin a fellowship in pediatric endocrinology at the University of California at San Francisco where he plans to pursue both his clinical interests in the management of diabetes and the metabolic syndrome, as well as his scientific interests in insulin signaling and insulin resistance. His career goal is to be an accomplished physician-scientist in the field of endocrinology at a major academic medical center.

Dr. Bremer is married to Dr. Daphne Carlson-Bremer, a veterinarian who will pursue her clinical and scientific interests in wildlife and conservation medicine when they move to California in 2005. Together they enjoy ballroom dancing, athletics, and outdoor activities.

Bryan H. Goldstein, M.D.

Dr. Bryan Goldstein obtained his B.A. in Law, Jurisprudence, and Social Thought from Amherst College where he graduated *magna cum laude* in 1999. After a brief stint as a chef, where he received the Certificate in the Culinary Arts degree from Boston University's School of Hospitality in 2000, he returned to academics at the Boston University School of Medicine. Dr. Goldstein received his M.D. degree from Boston University in 2004, where he graduated *magna cum laude*, and was elected to Alpha Omega Alpha in his junior year. He was also named the recipient of the 2004 School of Medicine and Boston Medical Center Department of Pediatrics Stephen R. Preblud, M.D. Memorial Award for Pediatrics.

In June 2004, Dr. Goldstein began his internship in pediatrics at the Boston Combined Residency Program in Pediatrics, which serves both Boston Medical Center and Boston Children's Hospital. He plans on pursuing a fellowship in pediatric cardiology at the completion of his residency. Dr. Goldstein and his wife Jaime were married in 2004, prior to the start of Dr. Goldstein's residency training.

Milton H. Nirken, M.D.

Dr. Milton Nirken obtained his B.A. degree *cum laude* in Biological Sciences from Rice University in 1962 and subsequently his M.D. degree from the Baylor College of Medicine in 1966. He did his pediatric residency at the Texas Medical Center in the Baylor College of Medicine Pediatrics Residency Program, and served as Chief Pediatrics Resident at Texas Children's Hospital in 1968.

In 1969, Dr. Nirken became Regional Chief of Pediatrics in the United States Air Force, and was stationed at Eglin Air Force Base in Florida. He then returned to Houston in 1971 and was a private practitioner for 22 years. While in the private sector, Dr. Nirken was a Clinical Associate Professor of Pediatrics at the Baylor College of Medicine, and since 1993, he has been a full-time faculty member of the Department of Pediatrics at the Baylor College of Medicine as an Associate Professor.

Dr. Nirken has been instrumental in establishing an Acute Treatment Area at the Texas Children's Hospital for ambulatory pediatrics, and at present is a full-time hospitalist at Texas Children's Hospital. He has completed a Master Teaching Fellowship Program at Baylor in 1997, and has also received the Pediatric Award for excellence in teaching from the Department of Pediatrics at the Baylor College of Medicine. Dr. Nirken has authored several articles in pediatric journals, and has more recently contributed to the establishment of the UpToDate in Pediatrics® Internet database.

About the Editor

Samir P. Desai, M.D.

Dr. Samir Desai serves on the faculty of the Baylor College of Medicine in the Department of Medicine. Dr. Desai has educated and mentored both medical students and residents, work for which he has received teaching awards. He is an author and editor, having written ten books that together have sold over 70,000 copies worldwide.

Dr. Desai is the author of the popular *101 Biggest Mistakes 3rd Year Medical Students Make And How To Avoid Them,* a book that has helped students reach their full potential during the third year of medical school. In the book, *The Residency Match: 101 Biggest Mistakes And How To Avoid Them,* Dr. Desai shows applicants how to avoid commonly made mistakes during the residency application process. He is also the editor of the

Clerkship Mistakes Series, a series of books developed to help students perform at a high level and acquire the skills needed for a successful career as a physician.

Dr. Desai conceived and authored the Clinician's Guide Series, a series of books dedicated to providing clinicians with practical approaches to commonly encountered problems. Now in its third edition, the initial book in this series, the *Clinician's Guide to Laboratory Medicine,* has become a popular book for third year medical students, providing a step-by-step approach to laboratory test interpretation. Other titles in this series include the *Clinician's Guide to Diagnosis* and *Clinician's Guide to Internal Medicine.*

In 2002, he founded www.md2b.net, a website committed to helping today's medical student become tomorrow's doctor. At the site, a variety of tools and resources are available to help students tackle the challenges of the clinical years of medical school.

After completing his residency training in Internal Medicine at Northwestern University in Chicago, Illinois, Dr. Desai had the opportunity of serving as chief medical resident. He received his M.D. degree from Wayne State University School of Medicine in Detroit, Michigan, graduating first in his class.

Foreword

Medical students enter their core pediatrics clerkship at different stages in their medical school careers. Some enter the clerkship directly following completion of the basic science portion of their curriculum; others already have experienced core clerkships in medicine, surgery, obstetrics and gynecology or other disciplines. I have had the great personal pleasure of teaching pediatrics to medical students and residents for more than forty years and repeatedly have heard comments at the conclusion of a clerkship from students that they had not anticipated the extraordinary differences between pediatric and adult care. Differences that they frequently delineate include: 1) the much greater need for reliance on parents or other family members for elucidation of a complete history; 2) the extent to which simple observation of the patient repetitively over time can help to elucidate the cause of an illness; 3) the rapidity with which the condition of a child can deteriorate or improve; 4) the necessity for having precisely the correct type of equipment; 5) the need for extraordinary specificity in formulation of fluid and electrolyte recommendation and medication dosages; and 6) the importance of the patient care team including nursing, pharmacists, physical and occupational therapists, child life play therapists, and others in affecting the optimal outcome for any given patient.

The primer which Drs. Bremer, Goldstein, Nirken, and Desai have authored incorporates all of these concepts and delineates, for the student, the optimal manner in which they can become an active participant in the patient care team, while concomitantly learning the basic fundamentals of pediatrics in a relatively abbreviated (approximately two months) period of time.

The authors have chosen to take the approach of listing statements which they believe to be in error and then defining the ways in which the student can avoid mistakes which can impact adversely upon the learning situation and upon their performance and enjoyment of the clerkship.

The authors also include a series of appendices that include excellent tips for success, helpful comments concerning interpretation of pediatric chest radiographs, and, a description of the more commonly employed infant and pediatric formulas as well as oral rehydration solutions.

I believe that this handbook would be of benefit to any student on any clerkship, because many of the points made within are applicable to both pediatric and non-pediatric clerkship experiences. The authors should be commended for taking the time to extrapolate from their own experiences to produce a text that would benefit every student immensely.

Ralph D. Feigin, M.D.
Chairman, Department of Pediatrics
Distinguished Service Professor
J. S. Abercrombie Professor of Pediatrics
Baylor College of Medicine

Physician-in-Chief
Texas Children's Hospital

Editor-in-Chief
UpToDate in Pediatrics®

Preface

My colleagues and I designed and wrote this book with one goal in mind—to improve the Pediatrics Clerkship experience for you, the medical student. And, throughout its development, we created a text that not only combines essential and difficult-to-find information, but also serves as a user-friendly guide through the multiple facets of pediatric medicine.

Unlike other Pediatrics Clerkship texts, this book is unique in that it takes you step-by-step through the daily activities of the Pediatrics Clerkship—whether on the inpatient wards, the outpatient clinic, or the nursery—and identifies mistakes commonly made along the way. The field of pediatrics is extensive, and medical students have a relatively brief period of time to learn its basic tenets. However, by reading this book, you will quickly gain an enhanced familiarity with the "nuts-and-bolts" of the Pediatrics Clerkship, and be well-prepared—even before setting foot in the hospital—for how to (i) excel during prerounds, work rounds, call, and attending rounds, and (ii) master write-ups, oral case presentations, and daily progress notes.

In this book, we identify 101 mistakes medical students commonly make during their Pediatrics Clerkship—all of which tend to negatively impact their overall experience. Then, after defining each mistake, we not only offer practical suggestions for how to avoid the error, but moreover provide specific instructions for how to become adept in the specific area of pediatric medicine in which the mistake was originally made. In this manner, our intent is to have you—the reader—learn from the mistakes of others—and avoid making the same or similar mistakes yourself.

Our desire is that after reading this book, you will have no "surprises" during your Pediatrics Clerkship and be well-equipped to gain the most from your experience. As we mention in the text, there is comfort in knowledge, and we hope that the information and insight this book imparts upon you will make you more content in the pediatric arena. Even more so, we hope that the knowledge you gain from this text will further your education and expand your clinical acumen and skills—in all areas of medicine.

Andrew A. Bremer, M.D., Ph.D.

Chief Resident, Internal Medicine-Pediatrics
Baylor College of Medicine

Acknowledgments

We would like to acknowledge the faculty members from the Departments of Pediatrics and Internal Medicine at the Baylor College of Medicine for their dedication to medicine and the education of physicians-in-training. We would also like to acknowledge our families—without whose support this endeavor would not have been possible.

Part I

Commonly Made Mistakes In

The Inpatient Environment

The majority of your time during your Pediatrics Clerkship will be spent in the inpatient arena; however, as pediatrics is mostly an outpatient specialty, the Pediatrics Clerkship will often incorporate several hours of clinic time per week—even during inpatient months. During your pediatrics inpatient experience, you will usually be part of a team responsible for the care of patients on the general medical floor or in the nursery. As in your other inpatient rotations, the medical team will usually consist of the following individuals:

Attending physician

The attending physician is typically a clinical or academic faculty member at the medical school who has been assigned to be the leader of the team. The attending physician's primary goal is to ensure that the patients assigned to the team receive the best possible medical care. Providing a solid educational experience for residents, interns, and medical students is another important role. The attending physician is also responsible for evaluating all the team members. The team's contact with the attending physician is usually limited to attending rounds, a period of time during the day in which the entire team meets with the attending. However, many attending physicians will also arrange lectures to be given explicitly for the medical students during the rotation.

Resident

The resident physician is the house officer who is responsible for overseeing the care of all the patients on the service. The resident has completed an intership and may have other clinical experience as well. The resident is responsible for overseeing the care of all the patients on the service. The resident supervises the work of the interns and medical students, and ensures that the treatment plans for the individual patients are implemented. The resident is also responsible for teaching the junior members of the team. Resident teaching may include didactic lectures, the demonstration of procedures, or pimping. For pediatrics, as with most rotations, the extent to which a resident teaches depends on the individual as well as the service.

Intern

By definition, internship refers to the first year of residency training that follows graduation from medical school. Next to medical students, interns are the most junior members of the team. Interns are responsible for executing the treatment plan on their patients and for writing the medical orders and daily progress notes. They also are responsible for communicating daily with the family on the condition of the child.

You will probably have the most interaction with the intern, since he or she will also be following patients assigned to you by the resident. The intern will probably expect you to be responsible for writing the daily progress note on your patients, which he or she will have to addend and cosign before it is entered into the permanent medical record. Some institutions permit medical students to write orders which then need to be cosigned by a physician before the order is executed. Other institutions will only permit orders to be written by physicians. When issues arise in the management of your patient's condition, you should always notify the intern immediately. However, if the intern is not available, notify the resident. The team will appreciate you keeping them informed of any issues regarding your patients. Although interns love to teach, this is not always possible given the demands placed upon them. On a daily basis, some of their responsibilities include scheduling tests or procedures, drawing blood or performing other procedures, checking lab test results, entering orders, writing daily progress notes, and communicating with patients' families.

On the inpatient service, here's what a typical day on the pediatrics rotation may look like:

7:00—8:00 AM - Prerounds
8:00—9:00 AM - Work-rounds

9:00—10:00 AM - - - - - - - - - - - - - Morning report or time
                                          to get your work done
10:00—12:00 NOON - - - - - - - - - - - - - - Attending rounds
12:00 NOON—1:00 PM - - - - - - - - - - - - Noon conference
1:00 PM—??- - - - - - - - - - - - - Time to get your work done
                                          (+ student conferences)

If you are not on call, the typical day ends about 5 PM.

In the text to follow, mistakes are discussed that are commonly made by medical students (1) during prerounds, (2) during work rounds, (3) while on call, (4) on write-ups, (5) on the oral case presentation, (6) on the daily progress note, and (7) during attending rounds.

Chapter 1

Commonly Made Mistakes During

Prerounds

During the inpatient portion of your pediatrics clerkship, your day will typically begin with prerounds. Prerounds refers to the period of time before the more formal rounding process with the entire pediatrics team. During prerounds, you will see your patients one on one or, occasionally, with an intern. The goal of prerounds is to identify new events that have occurred in your patient's course, record vital signs, fluid management and physical examination data, and assess the overall clinical status of the patient. The information you gather will be presented to the team during work rounds. The team typically consists of at least one resident, several interns, and an attending pediatrician. In this chapter, we will discuss commonly made mistakes during prerounds.

Mistake **#1**

Not knowing what to do during prerounds

Successful prerounding requires that you complete a set of tasks, as follows.

What to do during prerounds

- Review the chart for new progress notes that may have been placed since you left the hospital. This includes following up on outstanding consults, which may not be in the progress note section of the chart.

- Review the patient's orders, especially those for fluids and medications. Look for new orders, as changes that occur in the patient's hospital course are not necessarily documented in progress notes.

- Talk with the cross-covering intern who was taking care of your patient overnight to see if any new events occurred. If this is not possible, be sure to touch base with your intern, who should get sign-out from the cross-covering intern.

- Talk with the nurse who was involved in your patient's care to see if they have any concerns about the patient. In pediatrics, the nurses are an important source of information, particularly if the patient's family is not available.

- Talk with the patient's family to see if they have any concerns or questions regarding the care of the patient. In pediatrics, the patient's parents are often the only ones who know how the child is feeling. You should try to ascertain the following:

  ☐ Has the patient's overall condition improved, stayed the same, or worsened?

  ☐ Does the patient still have the same symptoms? If so, have the symptoms improved, stayed the same, or worsened?

  ☐ Does the patient have any new symptoms?

  ☐ Does the patient have any new concerns?

- If the patient can carry on a conversation with you, talk with him or her. Although most children are exceedingly shy around strangers, particularly physicians, sometimes the child will tell you something they didn't even tell their parents. Ask the child the same questions you asked the parents, above.

- Examine the patient. You should do the following:

☐ Write down vital signs, including weight.

☐ Pay particular attention to I/O's (I's = everything the patient has taken in by mouth/IV/NG, O's = everything the patient has put out in urine/stool/emesis/NG tube/ other tubes or drains). Be sure to keep track of the individual data—how much was put out as urine vs. JP drain, for example—as knowing only the cumulative output value often times is not helpful.

● Perform a brief physical examination: examine the areas of interest. For example, if the patient has a foot ulcer, take a look at the foot! At the minimum, you should perform a HEENT (head, ears, eyes, nose, and throat), heart, lung, abdominal, and extremity examination, irrespective of the complaint which led to the hospitalization.

Mistake #2

Setting aside too little time for prerounds

The amount of time needed for effective prerounding will depend on many factors, some of which include the following:

● The number of patients you are following

● The complexity of the patient's problem(s)

● The involvement of the family in the patient's care

Early in the rotation, you may require more time per individual patient to complete the preround tasks. However, your efficiency will improve as you become more familiar with the patients, the hospital, and your responsibilities.

Success tip #1

As a general rule, give yourself around twenty minutes to preround on each patient. That way, you will have enough time to complete the data gathering tasks noted above as well as formulate a coherent assessment and plan.

Mistake #3

Not having the proper equipment with you

Each specialty has unique tools of the trade such as bandage scissors for surgery and a pregnancy wheel for OB/Gyn which are integral to proper patient care and necessary for efficient and thorough prerounding. For pediatrics, you should have the equipment listed in the following box readily available:

Equipment needed for effective prerounding

Stethoscope (with pediatric bell and diaphragm, if available)
Otoscope/ophthalmoscope
Calculator
Reflex hammer
Measuring tape (have a few disposable pediatric measuring tapes, if you can find them)
Tongue blades
Penlight or flashlight

Success tip #2

Have a toy handy—in the pocket of your laboratory coat or near the equipment you'll be using—to distract apprehensive children.

Success tip #3

Have fun stickers in your pocket so you can give patients a sticker after you examine them or perform a procedure on them.

Mistake **#4**

The medical record is not reviewed for new orders and/or progress notes during prerounds

The medical record (the patient's chart) is the vehicle through which the patient's care and status are documented during the patient's hospitalization. As the medical student, you will most likely not be directly informed of events that happened to your patient while you were out of the hospital. However, by quickly reviewing the orders and progress notes sections of the chart, you can familiarize yourself to the best of your ability with any major events that may have affected your patient while you were out of the hospital.

Success tip #4

Contact the cross-covering intern early in the morning during prerounds to ask if any significant events occurred to your patients while you were out of the hospital. Often the cross-covering intern will be able to share more information with you regarding the status of your patients than he or she was able to document in the chart.

Mistake **#5**

The status of the patient is not discussed with the patient's nurse(s) during prerounds

As with all inpatient medicine, it is often the nurses who are most familiar with how the patient is doing, and know whether or not all aspects of the patient's treatment plan are being implemented. Be sure to touch base with the nurse(s) taking care of your patient during prerounds, and specifically ask them if any notable events occurred while you were out of the hospital. As stated above, nurses are an invaluable source of information on the pediatric wards, especially if the patient's family is not available for consultation.

Success tip #5

Be friendly to the nurses taking care of your patients and treat them with the same pleasantness and respect that you expect for yourself. A little common courtesy can go a long way toward building trust with your fellow caregivers.

Mistake #6

The status of the patient is not discussed with the patient's family during prerounds

As alluded to above, interacting and communicating with the patient's family is integral to proper patient care in pediatrics. More often than not, the family knows more than the nurses regarding the patient's status. It is also common for the pediatric patient to be unable or not want to fully communicate his or her feelings and needs to the medical team. For these reasons, it is imperative that you ask the child's family how the child is doing so that the team can provide effective patient care.

Mistake #7

A focused physical examination is not performed

Despite all the technology that is available in today's medical environment, the importance of the bedside physical examination must not be overlooked. Your resident and intern will expect you to physically lay hands on your patient every morning. Your patient is likely to be sleeping early in the morning during prerounds, but it is still imperative that you perform a focused physical examination.

Success tip #6

If your patient and one or more parents are sleeping, gently awaken the parents first and inform them that you are going to examine their child. Then proceed to awaken the child and complete the physical examination. By alerting the parents first, you will avoid the possibility of their being awakened abruptly by the cry of their child during the physical examination.

Success tip #7

Inform the older pediatric patient of what you are going to do during the physical examination before you do it. For example, before you lift up the gown tell the patient that you would like to listen to his or her heart.

Success tip #8

For patients who are old enough to understand, ask how they feel they are doing while you are performing the physical examination. That way, if they feel something is not going well, you can address it then and there while you're physically present.

Success tip #9

In addition to performing a general physical examination, be sure to specifically examine any part of the body for which the patient is being hospitalized. For example, if the patient is hospitalized for an abscess of the right foot, be sure to examine the right foot every morning.

Success tip #10

For certain diseases, it is important to note the time of your examination in relation to when the patient is receiving treatments for their disorder. For example, if a child hospitalized for asthma received his or her albuterol treatment 10 minutes prior to your examination, the lungs may sound clear with no expiratory wheezing. However, in two hours during work rounds, the pulmonary examination may have changed dramatically. The best way to document your examination would be as follows:

"Lungs clear to auscultation with no expiratory wheezes - 10 minutes post-albuterol therapy."

Mistake #8

The information obtained from prerounds is not written down in an organized fashion

Although you may have a great memory, write down pertinent information in an organized manner so that it is readily accessible. Examples of pertinent patient information include the patient's name and medical record number, date of admission, admission diagnosis/ diagnoses, daily vital signs, abnormal physical examination findings, abnormal laboratory values, diagnostic imaging results, and medications. These can be written on an index card or entered into a palm pilot for efficient recall. In so doing, you will not only keep better track of your patients but also have a quick reference to pertinent patient information.

Success tip #11

Organize the information gathered from prerounds in such a way that it can be easily accessed and conveyed to the team during work rounds.

Success tip #12

Document the patient's chronological age and, for preterm newborns, corrected post-gestational age; weight in kilograms; percentile with respect to height, weight, and head circumference (if less than two years of age); and BMI. The patient's age and weight should be recorded during prerounds every day. The percentile with respect to height, weight, head circumference (if less than two years of age), and BMI can be recorded on a weekly basis.

Mistake #9

The patient's vital signs are not recorded during prerounds

As in all areas of medicine, the pediatric patient's vital signs are integral to the interpretation of the patient's overall health and well-being. Unfortunately, documentation of the patient's vital signs is often inadvertently omitted during prerounds. Retrieving the vital signs, which are often recorded on a bedside flow sheet, is sometimes difficult during prerounds, since this time of day (about 7:00 AM) often coincides with changes in nursing shifts and nursing sign-out. Nevertheless, make every effort to obtain this information.

Success tip #13

Always ask the nurses taking care of your patient if
there were any aberrant vital signs recorded
overnight—particularly with respect to the patient's
temperature (fever).

Success tip #14

At the beginning of the rotation, ask the nurses taking
care of your patient where the vital sign information is
recorded. That way you will know exactly where to
look for it every morning during prerounds.

Success tip #15

When recording the patient's vital signs, record the
patient's T_{max} (maximum temperature over the
preceding 24 hours), T_c (current temperature), and
current value and 24-hour ranges for: heart rate,
respiratory rate, blood pressure, O_2 saturation, and
finger stick glucose (when appropriate).

Mistake #10

Not knowing how to document your patient's ins and outs

Although ins and outs in adult medicine are usually
documented in terms of mL/day, these absolute numbers
are often difficult to interpret in pediatric medicine since
the adequacy of these numbers depends upon the
weight and size of the pediatric patient. For example, an
intake of 1500 mL would be interpreted much differently
for a 25 kg child than for a 10 kg child, as would an output
of 1500 mL.

Fluid balance is very important in the management of
pediatric patients, especially neonates, and knowing the

exact ins and outs for your patient is information that will be requested during work rounds and is important for proper patient care. Document the patient's ins in terms of both total volume (mL's or liters/day) and volume adjusted for weight (mL/kg/day). The outs should be recorded in terms of both total volume (mL's or liters/day) and hourly volume adjusted for weight (mL/kg/hour). The patient's ins will consist mostly of IV fluids and enteral nutrition; the patient's outs will be comprised primarily of urine output and stool. However, other ins and outs are possible. For example, in a 6 kg patient, you might note:

"Ins = IV fluids (D10W + NaCl 2 mEq/100mL + KCl 2 mEq/100mL) @ 80 mL/kg/day + PO formula (Enfamil 20®) @ 20 mL/kg/day for total of 100 mL/kg/day or 600 mL/day; outs = urine output (UOP) @ 3 mL/kg/hour + 2 stools for total of 432+ mL's over 24 hours."

Success tip #16

Have a calculator with you and accessible during prerounds so you can quickly calculate the patient's ins in term of mL/kg/day, and their outs in terms of mL/kg/hour.

Mistake **#11**

Not knowing the type of nutrition your patient is receiving

Nutrition in pediatric patients is very important. Knowing what types of nutrition (breast milk, formula, cereal) the patient is receiving is vital to comprehensive patient care, especially in neonates and infants.

It is also important to know the exact route of nutritional input, as some children may be receiving nutrition via non-traditional routes. Examples of enteral nutrition routes (nutrition that is delivered to the gut via various means) include by mouth (PO), oral-gastric (OG) tube, naso-gastric (NG) tube, percutaneous endo-gastric (PEG) tube, and gastric-button/tube (G button/tube).

Children who cannot be offered some or all of their nutrition enterally (via the gut) will typically be supplied with parenteral nutrition. Examples of parenteral nutrition include glucose-containing IV fluids, partial parenteral nutrition (PPN), and total parenteral nutrition (TPN). Total parenteral nutrition is typically broken down into distinct components with goals set for total calories, carbohydrates, amino acids, lipids, and an assortment of essential vitamins and minerals. The line-by-line TPN/ PPN ordering process is complex and institution specific, and beyond the scope of this text. A lecture or review session with a pediatric nutritionist or dietician is often included in the curriculum of the clerkship.

Success tip #17

Document during prerounds the specific diet your patient is receiving, including its rate of administration and route of delivery, as this information will be requested of you during work rounds. If the diet is anything other than regular, know the reason why. Often the type and route of nutrition a patient is receiving can be directly tied into the underlying diagnosis.

Mistake **#12**

Not knowing and documenting the medications your patient is receiving

It is important to know exactly what medications a patient is receiving in the hospital. This is true for both scheduled medicines and PRN (as needed) medications. You will often have to look at the nurses' "kardex," also known as the medication administration record (MAR), to know exactly which medications were or were not given and when. Be sure to locate the kardex during the inpatient aspect of your clerkship. In some hospitals, this information is now available on the computer. It is also important to know the route by which the medications are being given (IV or PO). Moreover, be sure to document whether or not a patient has drug allergies. Verifying that ordered medications were or were not given is important in evaluating the effectiveness of the therapeutic plan put forth by the medical team. On a daily basis during prerounds, document exactly which pharmacological agents your patient did or did not receive.

Success tip #18

Document each of your patient's medications by drug name, dose in total mg as well as mg/kg or mg/kg/day for medicines dosed more frequently than once a day, route, and frequency. For example:

"Amoxicillin 400 mg PO tid (= 40 mg/kg/day divided tid = 13.3 mg/kg/dose tid, for a patient weight of 30 kg)."

Success tip #19

If a medication was not given to your patient as scheduled, know the reason why. You will probably need to track down the patient's nurse to find out why the medication was withheld. Then it is important that you relay this information to the intern or resident. Believe it or not, a lot of useful information is gathered this way. For example, If you learn from the nurse that the scheduled promethazine was not given because the patient was not nauseous and was difficult to arouse, tell your intern or resident so that the patient's dose of promethazine is decreased, changed to a longer-interval dosing schedule, or made "prn."

Success tip #20

If a medication your patient is receiving has a pre-determined treatment course, such as a 14-day course of an antibiotic, make note of what treatment day the patient is on, and when the course is scheduled to finish.

Mistake #13

Not knowing why your patients are receiving the medications they are receiving

Although as a medical student you will most likely not be directly prescribing medications to your patients, recognizing the reasons why your patients are on certain medications will help you more fully understand the pathophysiology of the disease process and the patient's treatment plan.

Success tip #21

Review and understand the pharmacological basis for the medications prescribed to your patients.

Mistake **#14**

Not knowing age-appropriate values for vital signs, laboratory results, or imaging studies

In pediatrics, the interpretation of vital signs, laboratory results, and diagnostic imaging are all age-dependent. What may be acceptable for a 12-hour-old neonate may herald a catastrophic disease process in a 12-year-old child. Until you get a feel for what is normal for a given age range, consult a more experienced member of the medical team for help in interpreting vital signs, laboratory results, and imaging studies.

Success tip #22

Have a reference book such as *The Harriet Lane Handbook*® or *Riley's Kidometer*® available to look up age-appropriate vital signs and laboratory values.

Chapter 2

Commonly Made Mistakes During

Work Rounds

During work rounds, the entire pediatrics team, sometimes including the attending physician, will round on patients being covered by the service. This more formal rounding process (in comparison with prerounds, discussed in Chapter 1) is where the data gathered during prerounds is shared, assessments and plans are discussed and agreed upon, and often some teaching is performed. Rounds typically occur in one of the following two formats:

Sit-down rounds

> In this format the team will typically sit around a table and discuss each patient's care. This may include chalk-board style teaching but will not involve direct patient interaction.

Walk rounds

> This rounding style is less formal but takes more time because it involves the entire team walking from one patient's room to another, discussing each patient along the way. In this format, patient information is discussed in the hospital corridor, allowing for direct team interaction with the patient and the teaching of important physical examination findings.

In either scenario, the resident or attending physician will expect the most junior member of the team, who is following the patient, to present the patient on rounds.

After hearing the presentation, the team will discuss the patient's progress, any new events that have occurred, and formulate a treatment plan. In this chapter, we will discuss commonly made mistakes during work rounds.

Mistake #15

Not knowing your resident's expectations for you during work rounds

At the beginning of the rotation, ask the most senior resident on the team what he or she expects of you. It is best to know up front what your role and responsibilities as a medical student will be.

Success tip #23

At the beginning of the rotation, ask your resident the following five questions:

1. What time do work rounds begin?

2. Where do work rounds start?

3. How would you like me to present newly admitted patients during work rounds?

4. How would you like me to present old patients during work rounds?

5. How much time do I have to present patients during work rounds?

Mistake #16

Showing up late for work rounds

The prerounding process can be very busy, and unexpected things happen. However, if you show up late for work rounds because you spend too much time during prerounds, you slow down the entire team and put restraints on the amount of time dedicated to work rounds. When work rounds are delayed or prolonged, it is often the dedicated teaching time that is sacrificed.

Mistake #17

Not knowing how to efficiently present a patient during work rounds

The following approach provides a way of efficiently presenting a patient during work rounds.

The pediatrics work rounds presentation step by step

Step 1: Present the patient to the team by giving the patient's name, age, (post-gestational age, if appropriate), ethnicity, gender, and chief complaint or working diagnosis/reason for admission to the hospital. Note the hospital day, post-operative day, and antibiotic treatment day, when relevant.

Example: Amber Smith is a 10-day old, 40 2/7 week post-gestational age white female admitted to the hospital for a fever of unknown origin with a temperature of 101.2°F and dehydration. She is presently on hospital day #1, antibiotic day #1.

Step 2: Present the subjective data, which should include the patient's current status and any events/ complaints that have occurred or developed since the previous day's rounds.

Example: No new events occurred overnight. The parents state that the patient is now eating better and her fussiness has decreased.

Step 3: Present the objective data, beginning with the vital signs.

Example: Over the past 24 hours, the T_{max} was 99.8°F, and the T_C is 98.8°F. Current pulse is 125 beats per minute (bpm) with a range of 110-140 bpm, respiratory rate 40/min with a range of 30-40/min, blood pressure 85/ 45 mmHg with a range of 80-90/40-50 mmHg, and O_2 saturation greater or equal to 99% on room air. Weight today is 3800 grams—an increase of 20 grams from yesterday and an increase of just over 5.5% from her birth weight of 3600 grams. Ins were 100 mL/kg/day via IV fluids of D5 1/4 NS + KCl 2mEq/100mL for a total of 380 mL's plus breastfeeding PO ad lib; urinary output was 3 mL/kg/hour or 274 mL's over 24 hours, and the patient had 3 formed stools.

Step 4: Present the physical examination findings from your most recent examination. In addition to including the HEENT, heart, lung, abdomen, and extremity examination, also include findings pertinent to the patient's problems. Present both pertinent positives and pertinent negatives, but avoid presenting a laundry list of negative examination findings.

Example: Physical examination is notable for clear tympanic membranes bilaterally, a clear oropharynx, moist mucus membranes, clear chest, soft abdomen, skin without rashes, and well-perfused extremities.

Step 5: Present the laboratory test results. Include only new laboratory test results. Old results may be presented if needed as a reference point.

Example: All laboratory results this morning were normal. The HCO_3 was 24 mEq/L, up from 18 mEq/L on admission 24 hours ago. All CSF, blood, and urine cultures have been negative for 24 hours.

Step 6: Present the results of any diagnostic studies or imaging tests.

Example: Chest radiograph obtained yesterday revealed no infiltrates, effusions, or cardiothymic silhouette enlargement. The radiologist reported the film as normal for age.

Step 7: Discuss the problem(s) and treatment plan. The problems should be discussed in order of decreasing importance. Provide an assessment for each problem followed by the management plan.

Example: Problem #1 is fever of unknown origin. The patient has been receiving IV ampicillin and IV gentamicin since admission, and will continue to receive these IV antibiotics for at least 48 hours pending the results of her CSF, blood, and urine cultures. If the cultures come back positive, we will continue IV antibiotic therapy based on the identification and sensitivities of the pathogenic organism. If we continue IV gentamicin beyond 48 hours, we will also check serum levels to confirm appropriate dosing. If the cultures return without growth after 48 hours, we will discontinue the IV antibiotic therapy.

Problem #2 is dehydration. The patient has been breastfeeding well per her mother's report since admission and has also been receiving maintenance IV fluids. This morning her serum HCO_3 is normal and her examination suggests improved perfusion. The plan will be to decrease her IV fluid rate and strictly monitor her I/O's and daily weight. If the patient can breastfeed well enough to gain weight and maintain adequate hydration, we will discontinue her IV fluids.

Mistake #18

A to-do (scut) list is not made during work rounds

It is important that you remember to do everything requested during work rounds. Although you are the medical student, the intern and resident are relying on you to be a proactive physician for your patients. Remember to think of yourself as *the* responsible physician—with many layers of help should you need them for your patient.

Success tip #24

To avoid missing to-do items discussed during work rounds or brought up elsewhere, be sure to write down a list of tasks that need to be performed for each patient. Many students and residents choose to create such a list with small checkboxes preceding each item. You can then check off a box when that task has been performed. This way, nothing is missed.

Mistake #19

Orders are not written during work rounds

In most institutions, it is during work rounds that the care of each patient is most critically discussed and the day's plan established. Thus, getting orders written or entered during work rounds when it is early in the day and the plan is still fresh in mind allows for the most efficient model of care. Moreover, for students who need their written orders co-signed by a physician before they will be carried out, work rounds satisfies the criterion of having an intern or resident available. Keep in mind, however, the delicate balance between the need for practical and efficient delivery of care and the educational value found in the teachings offered during work rounds. If you are constantly busy writing the day's progress notes or orders during work rounds, you will be less likely to pick up on the lessons learned in the care of other patients with whom you are not directly involved. Some hospitals have addressed this dilemma by allowing the more senior residents to enter orders into a computer-based ordering system during work rounds, allowing the students and interns to fully participate in the ongoing discussions.

Success tip #25

Ask your intern and/or resident if you can write orders on your patient(s). Most public hospitals will allow medical students to write orders; however, the orders will not be executed until they are co-signed by a physician. Private hospitals may or may not allow this. Writing orders is a very useful learning experience. Writing orders in a clear and succinct manner (necessary to the proper execution of those orders) takes practice, and you will be a help to the team if you can demonstrate your ability to write medical orders properly.

Success tip #26

Carry blank order sheets with you on work rounds. That way, you will always have order sheets with you in case there are no more order sheets in the patient's chart (which is often the case), or the patient's chart is unavailable during rounds.

Success tip #27

If you are presenting a patient, ask another medical student or intern to write orders for you on your patient while your patient is being discussed. An alternative approach is to ask a student or intern to keep track of the suggested orders on a piece of scrap paper, allowing you to gain practice in writing orders on your patients after you finish presenting the patient.

Mistake **#20**

Not fully understanding the plan for the patient

Always make sure that you understand the plan for each patient as your intern will count on you to make sure the plan is carried out. If you have any questions regarding the care of a patient, it is always best to clarify them with the intern or resident before work rounds are completed and the orders entered. Realize that this suggestion has implications far beyond the proper execution of the intended medical orders. Understanding why a specific diagnostic laboratory test or study has been suggested and what the test entails are keys to strengthening and expanding your medical knowledge base.

Chapter 3

Commonly Made Mistakes While

On Call

Your time on call denotes the time frame during which you will be admitting new patients onto the pediatrics service. Traditionally, the time a pediatrics ward team is on call extends from 7:00AM on one day until 7:00AM the next day—although this may vary by institution and school. The thought of being awake or at the hospital for more than 24 hours while you are on call may be daunting to you as a medical student. Take courage in the fact that during your on-call time you will have opportunities to work up new, interesting patients and spend quality time with your team. In this chapter, we will discuss commonly made mistakes while on call.

Mistake **#21**

Being unfamiliar with your on-call responsibilities

When you are on call—or handling other responsibilities—always consult with the house staff at the beginning of the rotation to determine their expectations of you. In particular, ask them how many patients you are expected to admit while you are on call. Use the time you spend on call as a marvelous way to increase your autonomy with fewer nursing personnel and house staff around, compared to a week day with the same patient census. Thus you will typically have a greater degree of freedom and responsibility while on call. This can help develop tremendous confidence in the patient care setting, but it can also be frightening. While on call, it is vital that you know which intern or resident will be backing you up, and how to contact them (by beeper, usually) when needed.

Mistake **#22**

Not being adequately prepared for call

Despite spending the night in the hospital, you will be expected to be well-groomed and dressed in the morning when the rest of the pediatric team arrives. Most interns and residents have a designated "on-call bag" with extra clothes, scrubs, sweatshirt and sweatpants in case the call room is cold, a book, toothbrush, comb, towel, snacks, etc.

Success tip #28

Always bring your "on-call bag" with you on the first day of a rotation, or leave it in a nearby medical school locker, if available. Unfortunately, the call schedule for medical students is often not determined prior to the start of the rotation. However, if you bring your "on call" bag with you on the first day, you will always be prepared for the possibility of being on call that evening.

Mistake **#23**

Significant others are not contacted during on-call nights

With increased patient care responsibilities, call is often a busy time. However, it is the rare occurrence that you are *continuously* too busy to find the opportunity to call a significant other at home. Believe it or not, call nights are usually as tough (if not *tougher*) on your significant other, who is often alone at home, than they are on you. A short phone call will be appreciated and can help elevate both of your spirits.

Success tip #29

Leave your significant other a small present or note, at home, on your call nights. Little gestures such as these go a long way.

Mistake #24

Essential patient information is not obtained before the patient is seen

If you are contacted for a patient admission, be sure to obtain the patient's full name, medical record number, and hospital location. Also, be sure to notify your back-up intern or resident that you have been assigned a patient admission—even though they should have been notified already and often will be the ones contacting you about the patient in the first place.

Mistake #25

Gathering too much patient data prior to seeing the patient

While the house staff will typically get sign-out on a patient being admitted from the ER, or transferred from an ICU, do your best to avoid learning that information up front. The house staff gathers this information, often including laboratory data, in order to be more efficient in patient care. As a medical student, however, you need not be so efficient since you should not have an overwhelming amount of patient care responsibilities and will learn more by seeing the patient "blind." Imagine how your approach to a patient would differ, in terms of history taking and physical examination, if you already knew that the patient had a right lower lobe pneumonia and a history of immunodeficiency or if you knew that the patient was being admitted for hypoxia. Perform your history and physical examination without being overly influenced by conclusions arrived at by the ER physician. Determine which laboratory tests and imaging studies you would order, even though many of these tests will have been ordered already in the ER. Periodically, the ER diagnosis ends up being incorrect, and seeing the patient with an open mind allows you to generate a more appropriate differential diagnosis in the end.

Mistake **#26**

The patient is not seen in a timely fashion

The intern or resident will expect you to take the initiative in performing the history and physical examination in a timely manner unless an alternative arrangement has been made, such as the case of seeing the patient with an intern simultaneously. Although this differs by institution and school, the house staff often relies on the student to complete much of the paperwork that goes into an admission. Typically, the intern or resident will *also* complete admission notes, but yours will generally be the most lengthy and comprehensive. The sooner you see the patient and complete the admission note, with orders when needed, the sooner the initial plan for the patient can be implemented.

Mistake #27

Not knowing the approach to evaluating a new patient

The intern and resident will rely on you to perform a complete history and physical examination. *(To minimize repetition in the text, the components of the complete history and physical examination that need to be addressed when evaluating a new patient are discussed in detail later in the book in Mistake #39: Not knowing what to include in the write-up.)*

Unlike other areas of medicine, pediatrics is unique in that the medical caregiver (the pediatrician) is charged with caring for small, often nonverbal and non-communicating individuals, usually attached to one or more anxious adults—whose level of concern may or may not reflect the degree of health or illness of the child. Thus, in many respects, the practice of Pediatric Medicine, especially Neonatology, is more closely related to Veterinary Medicine than Internal Medicine! The evaluation of a pediatric patient therefore requires a close interaction not only with the patient, but also with the family and other caregivers. In evaluating the pediatric patient, it is the task of the pediatrician to (1) ascertain the needed information from the clinical history, which is usually offered second hand by the patient's family; (2) perform a physical examination on the child, who may be scared and fighting; (3) assess the condition of the child; and (4) formulate a therapeutic plan. This is what makes pediatrics fun and challenging! Listed below are some general tips to consider when taking and performing a pediatric medical history and physical examination.

History-taking tips

Tip 1: Attempt to have the entire family present when conducting the medical interview. Each family member may have something unique to contribute to the medical history or a variant perspective of the patient's illness. Also, different caregivers of the patient may have different recollections or thoughts about what may be wrong with the child, and why. Having everyone present at the same time during the medical interview permits the development of a consensus history and allows everyone to be on the same page regarding the patient's condition. Although gathering the patient's history from several individuals at the same time may appear to be a slow process, it usually is more efficient than taking the patient's history from each caregiver individually.

Tip 2: Be sure you understand the definitions of the terms the parents are using when describing the patient's symptoms. For example, "diarrhea" to a physician usually means increased quantity and discharge of semisolid or fluid fecal material—usually at least six times per day. On the other hand, one or two loose stools per day may mean "diarrhea" to a parent.

Tip 3: Use open-ended questions to initiate the history and ascertain the patient's symptoms, then transition to directive questioning to specifically qualify them. This is truly one of the most difficult to acquire skills of Pediatric Medicine, and it comes only with time and practice.

Tip 4: Be sure to include the patient in the interview. Although most of the time during the medical interview will be spent speaking with the patient's family (and most of the clinical information will be gathered from them), don't forget that the parents *aren't* the ones who are sick, and although they may like to think so, they *don't* always know everything about their child or their condition. If the child is old enough, engage them in the interview and ask them questions as well. You would be surprised just how precocious some children are!

Tip 5: Before finishing the interview, always ask something in the nature of *"Is there anything else that you would like to discuss or tell me before we move on...?"*

Tip 6: *LISTEN*—to the family and the child.

Physical examination tips

Tip 1: Form your general impression of the patient prior to starting the examination, as a child may become fussy and/or uncooperative once the physical examination has begun.

Tip 2: Do your best to keep the patient comfortable. Remember Piaget's stages as a helpful guideline. For an infant, consider examining the baby while she has a pacifier in her mouth or is in range of her mother's voice. For a toddler, think of examining the patient while she sits on her mother's lap. Or, for an adolescent female, attempt to auscultate the heart with the stethoscope under the patient's shirt, rather than asking her to remove the garment.

Tip 3: Always obtain the vital signs. However, if they have been recently recorded at the bedside, do not feel obligated to obtain a new set of values.

Tip 4: Always obtain height, weight, and head circumference (for patients less than two years of age). From these measurements, you will be able to document the child's percentile with respect to height, weight, and head circumference utilizing the appropriate growth chart or PDA program. This information will also help you calculate their BMI.

Tip 5: Consider performing the HEENT (head-ears-eyes-nose throat) examination *last,* as examining the child's ears and mouth will undoubtedly irritate the child. The head examination should include an assessment of the child's anterior and posterior fontanelles. Think of how this might help in assessing the overall volume status or in evaluating a patient where there is concern for hydrocephalus. When utilizing the otoscope for the ear examination, be sure to examine the tympanic membranes visually by observing them under a well-lit and magnified environment and dynamically by observing any motion of the tympanic membrane when pneumatic pressure is applied. A newborn eye examination is often limited to assessing for a red reflex that effectively evaluates for the presence of a retinoblastoma, but in an older patient, a full ophthalmologic examination is suggested.

Tip 6: In a young child (neonate, infant, toddler), consider initiating your examination with the cardiovascular and pulmonary components. These are two aspects of the examination which are negatively impacted, if not impossible to perform, once a child has become irritable.

Tip 7: When performing the pulmonary examination, do as much without your stethoscope as possible. Observe the child to assess the ease of their respiratory effort, looking specifically for the presence of nasal flaring, grunting, or retractions (which may be supraclavicular, suprasternal, intercostal, or subcostal in nature). Listen for an audible wheeze, whoop, or stridor—all of which may be heard without the use of a stethoscope.

Tip 8: When performing the cardiac examination, especially in newborns, it can be quite difficult to appreciate abnormalities as the heart rate is often greater than 150 beats/minute. Spend a few moments concentrating on each heart sound. As an example: Is S1 present and normal? Does S2 split physiologically, pathologically, or not at all? Is there a murmur, and, if so, is it during systole, diastole, or both? From where can the murmur be appreciated? The left heart border? apex? axilla? back?

Tip 9: When performing the abdominal examination, try to distract the child so that their abdomen remains soft. A soft abdomen is a requirement to assess for masses and organomegaly. Some methods of distracting an irritable patient include talking to the patient, turning on the television, or offering the patient some food or a toy. In older patients, bending the knees—and bringing the knees up off the examining table—can aid in relaxing a rigid abdominal wall.

Tip 10: Always inform the patient and family before performing the genital examination, and always ensure that a genital examination has been performed either by yourself, by another physician, or as a team. For a variety of reasons, the genital examination is uncomfortable both to pediatric patients and their parents. However, as with many other aspects of medicine, if you inform the patient and parents of your intentions prior to the examination even before the patient is completely undressed, you are less likely to run into difficulties.

Tip 11: In male patients, note whether both testicles are descended, as well as the position of the external urethral meatus, to evaluate for the presence of epi- or hypospadias. In female patients, note the condition of the vulva. Newborn girls can often have vaginal discharge soon after birth as a normal finding as the neonatal uterus received constant hormonal stimulation from circulating maternal hormones, only to be withdrawn abruptly when the umbilical cord was clamped. Neonatal breast tissue in males and females is also oftentimes found as a result of the same hormonal stimulation. In addition, note the patient's Tanner Stage and correlate the Tanner Stage to their chronological age.

Tip 12: In sexually active pediatric patients, look for the presence of urethral discharge or lesions suggestive of sexually transmitted diseases. Such findings, in addition to abrasions/bruises and other evidence of trauma, may also be present in younger non-sexually active patients who have been sexually abused or molested. *Always notify the intern or resident if anything looks suspicious in the genital area.*

Tip 13: The neurological examination is based primarily on your observation of the child. Watch to see how the child moves his or her head, eyes, and extremities. Also, depending on the age of the child, watch to see how the child crawls, walks, or runs. In the neonate, assess a number of basic reflexes including the Moro, suck, root, grasp, and fencing reflexes.

The goal of the pediatric physical examination is to be efficient yet complete, as many children will not tolerate a long examination. Don't worry if the examination takes a long time for you to complete at the beginning of the rotation, or if the child and parents become frustrated with your examination. As the clerkship progresses, your efficiency in performing the pediatric physical examination will improve.

Success tip #30

Talk with the patient and family while you are performing the physical examination, and explain to them what you are doing and why you are doing it, and what you plan to do next. That way, there are no surprises. For example:

"...now I'm looking into the ears to see if there is any evidence of a possible ear infection, and next I'll be looking in the throat..."

Such an approach will greatly increase patient and family comfort with you and, in turn, you with them. Many fears develop in the hospital because of unknowns. The more you can make the examination technique a "known" to the patient and family, the more comfortable they will be with your examination.

Success tip #31

To calm an anxious child when performing the ear examination, which is often the most difficult part of the pediatric physical examination, ask the child something like, *"Are there any bunny rabbits in your ears?"* as you are manipulating the otoscope.

Success tip #32

Always warm your stethoscope before placing it on the child's chest. A cold stethoscope may induce instant tears.

Success tip #33

If possible, attempt to obtain pertinent patient information from other sources such as the babysitter, nanny, or teacher. However, be sure not to breech the rules of patient confidentiality in the process. For example, when speaking with a patient's teacher or guidance counselor, it is acceptable to suggest that the student is a patient at your hospital, but it is unacceptable to speak of, or about, his or her specific diagnosis.

Mistake #28

The patient's medical records are not obtained or reviewed

As a medical student, your goal should be to know or have rapid access to as much information about the patients you take care of as possible. To do this, you will have to take a thorough history and perform a complete physical examination as discussed above, but there is often further medical information available about a patient. For those patients who have been admitted for hospital care previously, records were generated from that stay. Do your best to obtain those medical records—with consent from the patient or family if records need to be obtained from an outside facility—and take some time to review them. Attempt to understand any connections between previous hospitalizations and the current one. This process will be even more important when you are caring for a patient who is chronically ill.

Success tip #34

Always request that the patient's old chart be brought to the floor. This process has been made far simpler in those hospitals with access to electronic medical records.

Mistake #29

The ER or clinic notes are not reviewed

Unfortunately, it often takes hours for a patient to make it from the ER or clinic to the floor, and things happen along the way. As an example, a child with reported respiratory difficulties may appear quite stable on the floor, breathing comfortably without significant wheezing or retractions. However, it would be important to recognize that this child appears to be doing well because he or she has received continuous albuterol nebulizer treatments for an asthma exacerbation that initially presented just a few hours before in the ER. Alternatively, a young patient being admitted for a sepsis work-up may be afebrile according to vital signs taken on the floor. However, it would be key to know whether or not he or she was febrile on initial presentation to the clinic, and whether or not he or she received antipyretics or antibiotics prior to his or her arrival on the ward. Moreover, it is often the case that a child or family cannot fully articulate the admitting diagnosis for a variety of reasons, including fatigue, poor communication, lack of understanding of the medical system or pathophysiology of the underlying disease process, and others. Thus, a brief review of the ER data or clinic note may help you and the medical team—as well as the patient and family—understand the reason for admission as well as the diagnostic and treatment goals.

Success tip #35

Attempt to speak with the ER or clinic physician admitting the patient to the hospital in person or by telephone to ascertain their impression of the patient and plan for care. As a medical student, you will find that this aspect of patient care is often quite difficult, even frustrating, as most of the communication will take place between residents, with you simply getting sign-out second hand. When this occurs, use the lack of information to your advantage. Attempt to create your own differential diagnosis and diagnostic/ treatment strategy even though one may already have been developed in the ER. Being open-minded like this can pay off in helping to find an alternative or additional diagnosis or treatment strategy.

Mistake **#30**

A complete history and physical examination are not performed

See Mistake #27: Not knowing the approach to evaluating a new patient.

Mistake **#31**

Not thinking about your assessment and plan after evaluating the patient

Although you will discuss the patient with your intern or resident after you obtain a history and perform a physical examination and prior to presenting the patient on rounds and making major treatment decisions, it is always best to formulate an assessment and plan independently. In this manner, you will learn to think like a physician. This is your opportunity to reach beyond the world of scut work and following orders into the land of reasoning and rational thought. This is what makes doctors doctors, and why so many physicians are so passionate about what they do. If you have formulated an assessment and plan, when the intern and/or resident says to you *"...so, what would you like to do?"* you will have an idea—or more than one!—in mind. Don't be upset or frustrated if the resident disagrees with you, because at this point in your career you simply do not have the experience to be proficient at formulating the assessment and plan. What is important is that you have thought about your patient and integrated the various data points you gathered from the history, physical examination, chart review, and ancillary data into the most coherent and comprehensive assessment and plan that you are capable of creating at this time. Include a differential diagnosis ranked in order of likelihood, based on the data points you gathered and the disease prevalence of the diagnoses you are considering.

Mistake #32

Relying on your intern or resident to write the patient's admission orders

See one, do one, teach one is the mantra of the academic teaching hospital. Whether the activity is a lumbar puncture or the more mundane process of entering patient orders, you will learn more if you do it yourself. It is good experience and good practice for you to write admission orders on the patients you admit. Furthermore, in writing the orders, you will feel more actively involved in the patient's care, as you are acting as their primary in-house physician. In the following table, we have listed the components of the admission orders along with some suggestions and examples of what is typically written for each component. To remember the components of the admission orders, we like to use the mnemonic *ADC VAAN DIMLS*.

Writing admission orders

Component of admission order	Write...	Example
Admit to	Ward team Attending physician (include pager number) Resident (include pager number) Intern (include pager number)	Admit to Pediatric Ward Attending—Dr. Smith (beeper 1122) Resident—Dr. Jones (beeper 3344) Intern—Dr. Lakes (beeper 5566)
Diagnosis	Place condition/diagnosis that the patient is being admitted for, if known. It is also acceptable to place a symptom.	Diagnosis—diarrhea
Condition	Good/stable/fair/poor/guarded	Condition—stable
Vital signs	Per routine or q shift is usually sufficient for most patients on the general pediatrics ward unless the patient is unstable. For example, a child admitted for an asthma exacerbation or with seizures may require more frequent observation.	Vital signs—per routine
Activity	Bed rest/ambulate as tolerated. State whether or not the patient can leave the room and/or go to the playroom.	Activity—as tolerated
Allergies	List drug allergies here. If there are no drug allergies, write "NKDA," which stands for "no known drug allergies."	Allergies—penicillin, which causes rash

Nursing	Instructions for nursing should be placed here. These may include contact precautions for infectious diseases, strict I/O's, neuro-checks, finger-stick glucose measurements, special beds, incentive spirometry, nasogastic suctioning, checking feeding residuals, call intern or resident if…, etc.	*Nursing—strict I/O's, daily weights, strict hand washing after interacting with patient. Notify house officer for temperature > 100.4ºF.*
Diet	NPO/breastfeed/formula (specify which type)/clear liquids/refeeding diet/regular diet/constant carbohydrate diet, etc. In neonates, you will need to specify exactly how much and by what route the child is to eat (e.g., Enfamil 20 with iron, 100 mL/kg/day divided q3h, per orogastric tube).	*Diet—refeeding diet, PO ad lib*
IV fluids	Document the type and amount of IV fluids you want the patient to receive. (See Success tip #36).	*IV fluids—D5 1/4 NS + KCl 2mEq/100mL at 33 mL/hr (~100 mL/kg/day for 8 kg pt)*
Medications	Specify the medication as well as the dosage, dosage per kilogram, frequency, route of admission, and indication if the medication is a prn medication. For instance, if the child weighs 8 kg and you want to prescribe Ampicillin, write Ampicillin 800 mg IV q8h = 100 mg/kg/dose = 300 mg/kg/day divided q8h.	*Medications—Acetaminophen 120 mg (= 15 mg/kg/dose) PO q6h prn temperature > 100.4ºF*
Labs	Specify when and what type of laboratory tests should be ordered.	*Labs—Chem-7 and CBC with differential at first AM routine draw*
Special	Include anything else here that you haven't listed above, including any particular studies that need to be performed.	*Special—Send stool for rotavirus antigen.*

Success tip #36

As a general rule, IV fluids should be given to replace—

- Fluid deficit
- Ongoing losses (maintenance fluids)
- Sensible losses (NG tube residual, stool, urine)
- Insensible losses (sweat, respiration)

The fluid deficit may be easily calculated by assuming that any acute weight loss is due entirely to the loss of water weight. Thus, if a 10 kg child has been vomiting and having diarrhea for two days and presents to the ER weighing just 9 kg, it can be reasonably assumed that they have lost 1 kg, or one liter, of water. Their fluid deficit is, thus, 1 L.

Maintenance fluids may be approximated using the 4-2-1 rule or the 100-50-20 rule. To calculate maintenance fluids, utilize the following table, based on body weight:

Body weight	100/50/20 rule	4/2/1 rule
1-10 kg	100 mL/kg/day	4 mL/kg/hr
11-20 kg	50 mL/kg/day	2 mL/kg/hr
>20 kg	20 mL/kg/day	1 mL/kg/hr

The table above should be read as "additive." Thus, a 23 kg child would require maintenance fluids of 10 kg times 100 mL/kg/day or 1000 mL/day (first line), plus 10 kg times 50 mL/kg/day or 500 mL/day (second line), plus 3 kg times 20 mL/kg/day or 60 mL/day (third line), for a total of 1560 mL/day, or 65 mL/hr. This approximates very closely the result obtained using the 4-2-1 rule, which is 63 mL/hr. Typical electrolyte requirements, to replace ongoing losses (but *not* excessive losses, as seen in diarrhea or continuous emesis, etc.) are about 2-3 mEq/kg/day of sodium and 2 mEq/kg/day of potassium.

Example: IV fluids—D5 1/4 NS + KCl 2mEq/100 mL at 33 mL/hr (~100 mL/kg/day for 8 kg pt).

Mistake #33

Not notifying your resident when the patient is seriously ill or has had a change in their clinical course

It is *extremely* important for you to notify the intern and/or resident when your patient is seriously ill or when the clinical course has changed. Prompt communication is essential for proper patient care. Be sure to help out when your patient becomes less stable, but remember that those around you have more experience than you do.

Mistake #34

Discussing with the patient or family issues you are unsure of

As a student on the wards, you will spend a large amount of your day with a small number of patients. It is not surprising, then, that they will often consider *you* as the primary caregiver. You are therefore charged with the privilege and responsibility of providing counseling and guidance to the patient and family. This is what being a physician is all about! That being said, you will often be asked important medical—and non-medical—questions that may have a major impact on the various decision-making processes that occur around the patient's disease. You will have the answers to many of these questions. However, there will also be many times when you do not know the appropriate response or are not confident enough in your answer. In this case, it is always best to be honest with the individual who asked the question—deferring the response to a more senior member of the medical team. Particularly when it comes to questions of serious import, such as those with prognostic indications, it is best to allow those with more experience to speak with the patient or family, although you ought to be present to hear the response and learn from it. When faced with a question from a patient or family that you are unsure of, the best answer may be, *"I don't know, but I'll do my best to find the answer for you as soon as possible."* This is always an appropriate response.

Mistake #35

Not offering to help the team before leaving

Some medical schools do not require overnight call during the pediatric clerkship. Even if you are expected to spend the night, your intern or resident may give you the choice of going home. Regardless of the particulars of the clerkship or the pediatric team, it's always good policy to check in with your team prior to leaving the hospital. As a team player, offer your assistance for completing any unfinished tasks even if they aren't for your particular patients. While you might have to stick around for a few extra minutes on occasion, you will often be rewarded when others on the team look out for you at another time.

Success tip #37

Before leaving the hospital, make sure that all orders on your patients have been written and are being executed properly. Write orders for tasks that need to be performed prior to your return to the hospital the next day. For example, if a patient you are following needs a CBC drawn on the following day, write an order for *"CBC in AM (with the date noted)"* before leaving the hospital. Be sure the order is co-signed by a house officer.

Chapter 4

Commonly Made Mistakes On

Write-Ups

The written case presentation, or "write-up," is a detailed formal account of the patient's clinical presentation and illness. Although many students consider this task to be a bit tedious, developing the skills needed to document a patient's clinical course appropriately and comprehensively is essential in modern-day medicine. Effective written communication is a learned skill, and the ability to efficiently and succinctly document a patient's case is vital for communication between physicians and essential for delivering high quality patient care.

Mistake #36

Not understanding the importance of the write-up

The case write-up is an important task. Not only does it aid in the development of skillful written communication, but it also allows the student an opportunity to formally organize his or her thoughts and convey them in a clear and purposeful manner. This will, in turn, improve oral clinical presentation skills. Moreover, the write-up is an opportunity to make and see connections between the clinical presentation of symptoms and signs and the underlying pathophysiology of a disease process. The preparation for the write-up allows the student to delve deeper into the literature and understand more about specific diseases and diagnoses.

Mistake #37

The write-up is not turned in on time

The write-up should be presented to the intern, resident, or attending physician in a relatively short period of time, although the due date varies by institution. The goal of preparing the write-up is to generate a complete written version of the case history and clinical presentation. Timeliness should not win out over proper completion of the assignment, but by completing the write-up in a timely fashion, you will be more likely to receive constructive feedback before the deadline for subsequent patient write-ups. This feedback can then be utilized to improve upon the preparation of the next write-up, and your written case presentation skills in general.

Also, when you feel comfortable doing so, ask your reviewers for *specific* comments—positive and negative—regarding the quality of your patient write-ups. Settling for a "nice job" or "strong work" comment, while initially satisfying, offers little in the way of improving your written communication skills over the long term. Don't forget that the goal is to improve your career skills, a task much more important than enjoying a false sense of perfection on a given write-up. Realize that criticism does not suggest that a poor job was done. On the contrary, residents will recognize those students who want feedback beyond "great job" as those who truly want to improve their work and are not simply satisfied with the appearance of a good grade.

Success tip #38

Ask your intern, resident, or attending to make specific comments regarding the content and quality of your write-ups, and to make suggestions for improvement.

Mistake **#38**

The write-up is not complete

As in other rotations, your residents and attending physicians will expect the patient write-ups you do during the pediatric clerkship to be complete. They should also be comprehensive and reflect the thoroughness of your evaluation. Although the pediatric write-up may be shorter than those in other clerkships such as internal medicine due to a lack of significant medical and surgical histories, the pediatric write-up is unique in several respects. See Mistake #39, below.

Mistake **#39**

Not knowing what to include in the write-up

At the beginning of the rotation, determine from the intern, resident, or attending physician what should be included in the write-up. Some items may be individual preferences while others may be fairly universal. The standard content of the pediatric write-up is usually divided among elements listed in the following box.

Elements of the pediatric write-up

Patient identification
Source of information
Chief complaint / reason for admission
History of present illness (HPI)
Past medical history (PMH)
Past surgical history (PSH)
Immunizations
Medications
Allergies   continued...

> Family history
> Social history
> Neurodevelopmental history
> Review of systems (ROS)
> Physical examination
> Laboratory data / other studies (chest radiograph, ECG, etc.)
> Assessment
> Plan

Although most students at this point in their career will have learned how to complete a write-up either from a physical diagnosis class or from a previously completed clerkship, listed below is a step-by-step approach to completing a pediatric case write-up. Specific details regarding what to include in each step in the write-up are provided with a checklist of items you should address before proceeding to the next step. Each item in the checklist is a common mistake students make in their write-ups.

Step 1: Patient identification

Students often forget to identify their patient on the write-up. Be sure to include the patient's name at the top of the write-up unless you are given instructions not to do so.

Step 2: Source of information

After identifying the patient, be sure to document all sources of patient information and their reliability. Please note that documentation of the source of the patient information and history is especially important in pediatrics, as more often than not the history is given by someone other than the patient.

continued...

Not uncommonly, the history is taken from multiple individuals such as the patient's mother, father, school teacher, or babysitter. Moreover, the history may be either slightly or vastly different depending on which source you speak with—which is why you also need to assess the reliability of the information you are receiving. In addition, as in other areas of medicine, patient information can also be obtained from old records, clinic notes, ER notes, transfer notes, etc.

Before proceeding to Step 3, you need to identify the following:

- ☐ Source of the patient's history
- ☐ Reliability of the source

Step 3: Chief complaint or reason for admission

The chief complaint or reason for admission should be stated in the patient's or caregiver's own words, if possible, along with its duration.

Before proceeding to Step 4, be sure you have written down the following:

- ☐ Chief complaint/reason for hospital admission
- ☐ Chief complaint, in the patient's or family's own words
- ☐ Duration of the chief complaint prior to admission

Step 4: History of present illness (HPI)

The HPI begins with an opening sentence that contains the patient's age (post-gestational age, if appropriate) and ethnicity—which is important because many genetic and metabolic disorders have variable prevalence across distinct ethnic groups—as well as gender, relevant past medical history, and chief complaint. Following the opening statement, describe the story of the patient's illness in chronological order leading up to the time of admission. Be sure to include associated symptoms, pertinent positives and negatives, any similar illness in the family, any recent travel, any prior exposure to contagious diseases, and ways the illness is affecting the patient's quality of life. Evaluations performed by other physicians during the course of the illness prior to the hospitalization, including results of diagnostic testing as well as response to any given treatment, should be included at the appropriate chronological point.

Before proceeding to Step 5, be sure that the HPI has the following characteristics:

☐ The first sentence or paragraph of the HPI includes the patient's exact age, ethnicity, gender, relevant past medical history, and health status prior to the development of the chief complaint.

☐ Information is presented in chronological order using days prior to admission rather than the actual days of the week. For example, *"Cough started three days prior to admission"* rather than *"Cough started on Wednesday."*

☐ The patient's chief complaint or symptom is fully characterized. For pain, comment on onset, location, quality, severity, and exacerbating and relieving factors.

☐ Pertinent positives and negatives are included.

☐ The report includes significant information from the past medical history, social history, family history, and review of systems relevant to the patient's chief complaint or presenting problems.

☐ Information about evaluations performed by other physicians during the course of the illness prior to hospitalization, including results of diagnostic testing and response to treatment is included.

☐ Information about the patient's emergency room course, if applicable, is included.

☐ The report is free of any past medical history not relevant to the patient's current illness.

☐ Review of systems information not pertinent to the patient's current illness is not part of the report.

Step 5: Past medical history (PMH)

In the PMH, include a thorough listing of all previously diagnosed conditions, including any supporting data. For a past medical history of diabetes, you might include age at diagnosis, degree of blood sugar control, insulin requirements, and presence of end-organ damage. The PMH should also include the prenatal, birth, neonatal, feeding, and growth history. Information involving childhood illness and prior hospitalizations belong here as well.

Past Medical History	
Element of the PMH	**What to include**
Prenatal history	Number of previous pregnancies and their results Duration of maternal pregnancy Any maternal illnesses or complications during pregnancy (glucosuria, diabetes, pregnancy-induced hypertension, illnesses, toxemia, bleeding, etc.) Amount of maternal weight gain during pregnancy Any unusual maternal exposures during pregnancy (radiation, chemicals, drugs, etc.) Any medications (prescription or non-prescription) taken during pregnancy Duration and adequacy of maternal prenatal care Results of tests performed during pregnancy (e.g., amniocentesis) Time and type of movements fetus made in utero
Birth history	Date Place Weight Height Head circumference Type of presentation (cephalic, breech, etc.) Duration of labor Complications of labor (e.g., failure to progress) Type of delivery (normal spontaneous vaginal delivery [NSVD], Cesarian section [C/S], vacuum-assisted, forceps-assisted, etc.) Anesthetics used during labor
Neonatal history	APGAR scores Birth weight Any perinatal complications such as resuscitation at birth, cyanosis, parenteral nutrition, oxygen requirements, incubator stay, jaundice, rashes, infection, etc. Age at discharge Results of neonatal screening tests such as hearing screen, vision screen, newborn metabolic screen, etc.

Feeding history	How well baby took the first feeding If breast fed (partially, entirely, for how long, etc.) If formula fed (partially, entirely, amount/24 hours, type, need for any formula change, for how long, etc.) Age at weaning Typical feeding schedule When solids were introduced (and how they were tolerated) Any vitamin supplementation, including type (e.g., iron, vitamin D, fluoride), amount, date started, and duration Present diet (amount of cereal, vegetables, fruit, dairy, and meat) Any potential feeding problems (e.g., aspiration with thin liquids)
Growth history	History of height, weight, head circumference, and BMI with respect to national standards. In order to do this properly, you will need to have access to age- and gender-appropriate growth charts.
Past illnesses	Focus on infections (age, type, number, severity), contagious diseases (varicella, mumps, scarlet fever, etc.), accidents, and injuries
Prior hospitalizations	Include date, location, diagnosis, treatment, hospital course, complications, date of discharge, etc.

Before proceeding to Step 6, be sure that the PMH includes the following:

☐ All supporting data

☐ Prenatal history

☐ Birth history

☐ Neonatal history

☐ Feeding history

☐ Growth history

☐ Past illnesses, including common childhood illnesses

☐ Any prior hospitalizations

Step 6: Past Surgical History (PSH)

In the past surgical history, include any prior operations such as circumcision, procedures such as central line placement, umbilical line placement, etc., and any associated complications such as excessive bleeding. Also include head injuries, fractures, and other traumatic events.

Before proceeding to Step 7, be sure that the PSH includes the following:

☐ All past operations/procedures

☐ All past traumatic events, along with their dates

☐ Any associated complications with prior operations/ procedures

Step 7: Immunizations

Under immunizations, list all prior immunizations and their dates of administration. Include HBV, HAV, DTaP, Hib, IPV, PCV, MMR, varicella, and BCG. To correctly evaluate the immunization status of the patient, you will need to be familiar with standard age-appropriate immunizations as well as other vaccine recommendations applicable to patients with chronic medical conditions. Examples of such patients include those with HIV or sickle cell disease or other high-risk patient populations such as former premature infants or patients undergoing chemotherapy. Document any missing immunizations along with reasons why the immunization history is not up to date.

Before proceeding to Step 8, be sure that you have recorded the following:

☐ All immunizations the patient has received, the dates given, boosters, and complications

☐ Immunizations that the patient is lacking if the immunization history is not up to date

☐ Documentation of reasons why the patient is not up to date on immunizations

---

Step 8: Medications

In the medication section of the write-up, list all prescription and non-prescription medications the patient is taking, including over-the-counter (OTC) medications and herbal supplements. Don't forget to include the name, dose, frequency, and route of administration. Be sure to list the indication for all the medications as well.

Before proceeding to Step 9, be sure you have included the following:

☐ A list of all medications the patient is taking

☐ Indications for each medication

☐ Groupings of the medications given for the same condition

☐ Exact dosages of the medications expressed in milligrams (mg) or grams (g), amount/kg, and amount/kg/dose

☐ Route of medication administration (e.g., PO)

☐ Frequency of medication administration (e.g., bid)

☐ Any recent change in dose

☐ Discontinuation of any medication by the patient's physician, including the date of and reason for discontinuation

☐ List of any medications the patient is not compliant with

☐ OTC or herbal medications or supplements the patient is taking

☐ Do NOT include any new medications started in the hospital

Step 9: Allergies

List allergies to any medications, along with the *specific* reaction the patient had to the medication (e.g., allergy to sulfa drugs, which causes an erythematous rash). Remember that patients often state that they are "allergic" to a medication when, in fact, what they may have experienced was a side effect; thus, patients often unknowingly report expected side effects of a given medication as a medication allergy. For example, a patient may say they are allergic to morphine because it makes them nauseous. However, this is an expected *side effect* of the medication as opposed to an *allergic response* to the medication. Don't forget to list allergies to any foods, inhalants, or substances contacted directly such as poison ivy, betadine, or latex.

Before proceeding to Step 10, be sure you have documented the following:

☐ Allergies to any medications

☐ Reaction to medications the patient reports being allergic to

☐ Allergies to any foods, inhalants, or contacts

Step 10: Family history

In the family history, include any history of genetic and/or metabolic diseases (diabetes, hemoglobinopathies, cystic fibrosis, galactosemia, etc.), sudden, unexplained deaths (hypertrophic obstructive cardiomyopathy, prolonged QT syndrome, etc.), and communicable diseases such as tuberculosis. Ask your attending whether the information should be presented in a family tree or inheritance chart. Information about parents, siblings, and grandparents should be documented, including age, health status, and cause of death.

Before proceeding to Step 11, be sure you have completed the following:

☐ Constructed a family tree or inheritance chart

☐ Identified any family history of genetic disorders

☐ Identified any family history of sudden, unexplained deaths

☐ Identified any family history of communicable diseases

Step 11: Social history

What to include in the social history

People the patient lives with (parents, grandparents, aunts, uncles)

The patient's primary caregivers (mother, father, etc.)

The patient's other caregivers (babysitters, friends, etc.)

continued...

Education level of the patient's primary caregivers

Socioeconomic status of the patient's parents

Religious affiliation of the patient's parents (Jehovah's Witnesses, Catholic, etc.). This is important when it comes to the family's views on blood transfusions, birth control, etc.

Marital status of the patient's parents

Information regarding the patient's siblings (if applicable)

Where the patient lives (city, suburb, etc.)

Patient's type of living environment (home, condominium, apartment, mobile home, etc.)

Condition of the living environment

Year the living establishment was built/renovated (this is particularly important when it comes to leaded paint and the potential for lead intoxication)

Whether the patient attends day care or school, or is cared for at home

Whether the patient has had any sick contacts prior to his/her hospitalization

Whether any pets live at home with the patient (cats, dogs, reptiles, etc.)

Whether the patient uses alcohol, tobacco, or any other drugs

Whether the patient is sexually active (if applicable)

continued...

How the patient is doing in school (in particular, what types of grades and behavioral scores the patient is receiving)

Whether the patient is employed and if so, where the patient is employed and what type of work the patient is doing

Before proceeding to Step 12, be sure you have documented the following:

☐ Whom the patient lives with

☐ Where the patient lives, especially the living conditions

☐ Who the patient's caregivers are (parents, relatives, friends, babysitters, etc.), including their specific responsibilities, such as feeding the patient, babysitting on weeknights, or taking care of the patient on weekends

☐ Whether the patient attends day care or school or is cared for at home

☐ Whether the patient has had any sick contacts prior to their hospitalization

Step 12: Neurodevelopmental history

What to include in the neurodevelopmental history

Ages when the patient attained specific neurodevelopmental milestones (raising head, rolling over, smiling, maintaining a sitting position without support, walking with or without support, first words, first sentence, bowel and bladder continence, etc.)[*]

continued...

Whether the patient has lost any previously attained neurodevelopmental milestones

How the patient is doing in school (school performance and extracurricular achievement)

Involvement in extracurricular activities (sports, dance, language, etc.)

Personality (happy, easy-going, shy, etc.)

Behavior, including behavior with respect to siblings or peers and ability to get along with other children

Habits (tantrums, nailbiting, thumbsucking, etc.)

How the patient compares to his/her siblings (if applicable)

* To determine if the patient is developing "on track," you will need to familiarize yourself with the appropriate ages at which certain neurodevelopmental milestones are attained (see Appendix G: Age-Appropriate Developmental Milestones).

Before proceeding to Step 13, be sure you have documented each of the following:

☐ The ages at which the patient attained neurodevelopmental milestones including smiling, maintaining a sitting position without support, walking without support, first words, first sentence, and bowel and bladder continence

☐ The ages at which any attained neurodevelopmental milestones were lost (if applicable)

☐ How the patient is doing in school

☐ The patient's activities outside of school

☐ The patient's personality, behavior, and habits

Step 13: Review of Systems (ROS)

Review of systems element	What to include
General	Overall health, growth, and development including change in weight, appetite, activity level, and fatigue
HEENT	History of strabismus, glasses, eye infection, discharge, redness, visual problems, otitis media, hearing problems, vertigo, sore throat, rhinitis, snoring, dental abnormalities, choking with feeds
Respiratory	History of coughing, wheezing, hemoptysis, dyspnea
Cardiovascular	History of palpitations, cyanosis, fatigability, chest pain, shortness of breath, syncope, murmur, edema
Gastrointestinal	History of abdominal pain, colic, vomiting, diarrhea, constipation, hematochezia, melena, jaundice
Genitourinary	History of urinary tract infection, hematuria, enuresis, dysuria, frequency, polyuria, vaginal discharge, menstrual history (if applicable)
Musculoskeletal	History of joint abnormalities, arthralgias, arthritis, ligamentous laxity, muscle pain, limb-length inequalities, gait abnormalities, weakness
Skin	History of rashes, hives, skin discoloration, unusual skin pigmentation, swelling, change in skin color, problems with hair
Neurologic	History of convulsions, tics, weakness, headache, dizziness, mental status changes, disorientation
Psychiatric	History of changes in personality, unusual behaviors

Before proceeding to Step 14, be sure you that in the Review of Systems, you have remembered to document the following:

☐ How the patient is doing in general

☐ How the patient is eating

☐ How the patient is voiding

☐ How the patient is sleeping

☐ Whether or not the patient has lost or gained any weight. Document the amount and time period of weight change, when applicable.

☐ How the patient is progressing along his or her growth curves with respect to height, weight, head circumference, and BMI. In order to do this appropriately, you will need to have age- and gender-appropriate growth charts available.

☐ Do NOT repeat any review of systems documented in the HPI or elsewhere in the write-up.

Step 14: Physical Examination

Physical examination element	What to include
Vital Signs	Temperature, heart rate, respiratory rate, blood pressure (in upper and lower extremities, if necessary), and, if applicable, pulse oximetry and orthostatic vital signs.
Measurements	Weight, height, head circumference (up to 2 years of age), and BMI. Also include the patient's percentile with respect to height, weight, head circumference (up to 2 years of age), and BMI.
General	Patient's general appearance (well-nourished, mildly dehydrated, cachectic, etc.)

Head	Head shape (is there plagiocephaly?), fontanelles, sutures, presence of lesions, etc.
Eyes	Appearance of the eyes, visual fields, gross visual acuity (how well can the patient see?), palpebral fissures, function of the extraocular muscles, red reflex for newborns, size of the pupils (is there anisocoria?), reactivity of the pupils, strabismus, and fundus from the ophthalmoscopic examination.
Ears	Configuration of the ears, gross auditory acuity (how well can the patient hear?), any peri-auricular lesions such as pits or tags, external ear canals, discharge, tympanic membrane anatomy (light reflex), tympanic membrane motility (pneumo-otoscopic examination).
Nose	Nasal septum, turbinates, mucous membranes.
Throat and mouth	Lips, gums, tongue, teeth, oropharynx, palate, tonsils.
Neck	Presence of any masses, webbing, thyromegaly, cervical lesions (sinus tracts), lymphadenopathy, range of motion, torticollis, rigidity.
Chest	Symmetry, expansion, lesions (pectus deformities), breast development. Assess for gynecomastia in males and Tanner stage in females.
Respiratory	Lung sounds (wheezes, crackles, rhonchi), inspiratory/expiratory chest movement, use of any accessory muscles of respiration.
Cardiovascular	Dynamics of the precordium, point of maximum impulse, murmurs (systolic, diastolic, continuous), rubs, gallops, heaves, thrills, etc.
Gastrointestinal	Presence of tenderness or distension, whether the abdomen is soft or rigid, bowel sounds, organ size (is there organomegaly of the liver and/or spleen?), etc.

Genitourinary	Tanner stage of the genitalia. For males, comment on the location of the testicles and whether they are both descended into the scrotal sac, circumcision, hydrocele, hernia, and phimosis. For females, comment on the appearance of the genitalia (is there any vulvar irritation or vaginal discharge?), the vaginal orifice (is there an intact hymen?), hernia, and clitoral enlargement.
Anal / rectal	Presence of anal fissures, excoriations, rectal prolapse, hemorrhoids, etc.
Back	Comment on the curvature of the spine (is there lordosis, scoliosis, kyphosis?), costovertebral angle tenderness, dimples, or tufts of hair possibly indicating a spina bifida occulta.
Musculoskeletal	Peripheral pulses, active and passive range of motion, cyanosis, clubbing, edema, limb-length inequality, hemihypertrophy, muscle bulk.
Skin	Rashes, lesions (macules, patches, papules, nodules, pustules, etc.), discoloration, pigmentation, swelling, etc.
Neurologic	Mental status, cranial nerve function, motor function, sensory function, deep tendon reflexes, cerebellar function, spasticity, tremor, rigidity, clonus, etc.

Before proceeding to Step 15, be sure you have completed the following:

☐ Documented a *thorough* and *complete* physical examination. In addition to the above recommendations, refer to Mistake #27: Not knowing the approach to evaluating a new patient.

☐ Listed the patient's vital signs

☐ Actually listed the vital sign values rather than writing *"patient afebrile"* and *"vital signs stable"*

☐ Remembered to include orthostatic vital signs and pulse oximetry readings, if applicable

☐ Recorded the patient's percentile with respect to height, weight, head circumference (up to 2 years of age), and BMI

☐ Remembered to avoid making any judgments about physical examination findings in this portion of the write-up

---

Step 15: Laboratory data / other studies (chest radiograph, ECG, etc.)

Include official results of all laboratory data, imaging studies, and other diagnostic tests.

Before proceeding to Step 16, be sure you have completed the following tasks relative to diganostic studies:

☐ Documented the official results of all laboratory data, imaging studies, and other diagnostic tests

☐ Avoided interpreting data in this portion of the write-up

☐ Circled or highlighted abnormal values. In order to do this, you will need to know age-appropriate normative values for the data.

Step 16: Problem list

All significant problems or abnormalities identified in the database (history, physical examination, laboratory findings, etc.) should be listed in what is termed the "problem list." The problem list, which is written just before the summary statement, assessment, and plan, should be presented in a bullet point format.

continued...

Initially, your problem list may be quite long, but as you gain experience in synthesizing data from the history, physical examination, and laboratory data, you will be able to recognize relationships among some of the problems on the list. This will allow you to place them under one heading rather than multiple headings. Most important early in your career is the ability to identify all abnormalities.

Before proceeding to Step 17, be sure to do the following:

☐ Include a complete problem list

Step 17: Assessment/Plan

After reporting the history, physical examination, results of laboratory or diagnostic studies, and problem list, the assessment and plan begins with a summary of the patient's clinical presentation. The development of the summary is an exercise that requires you to focus on the most pertinent data in the patient's clinical presentation. It should be no longer than half a page, and include all the pertinent positives and negatives of the history, physical examination, laboratory data, and diagnostic studies.

After the summary, discuss each of the patient's problems in descending order of importance. For each problem, provide both an assessment and plan. In your assessment, include a differential diagnosis ranked in order of likelihood. For your working diagnosis, the diagnosis that best explains your patient's clinical presentation, explain your rationale. Discuss your reasoning and include diagnostic criteria for the working diagnosis. continued...

Support your conclusion with data, including elements of the history, physical examination, and laboratory and imaging data. Following the assessment, an organized plan should include other diagnostic studies needed to confirm your working diagnosis or exclude other conditions in the differential diagnosis. This should be immediately followed by the treatment plan.

While you should certainly use textbooks of pediatric medicine as well as current literature to help you construct the assessment and plan, be sure that your comments apply directly to your patient. The assessment and plan give you the opportunity to demonstrate your firm grasp of your patient's problems.

Before completing the write-up, check to be sure you have done the following:

- ☐ Included a summary statement
- ☐ Prioritized the patient's clinical problems
- ☐ Included an assessment for every problem
- ☐ Included a plan for every problem
- ☐ Created an assessment that includes a prioritized differential diagnosis, including common and potentially life-threatening conditions
- ☐ Provided support for your working diagnosis using information from the patient's history, physical examination, and laboratory, imaging, and other data
- ☐ Created a plan documenting further diagnostic studies needed to confirm the working diagnosis or exclude other conditions in the differential diagnosis if needed
- ☐ Documented a complete treatment plan along with your rationale

Chapter 5

Commonly Made Mistakes On

The Oral Case Presentation

As with written communication, effective oral communication is essential for good medical practice and proper patient care. However, proficiency in one aspect of medical communication does not ensure a similar level of skill in the other; it is important to master both forms of communication. Although similarities do exist between the case write-up and the oral case presentation, the oral case presentation in general serves a much different purpose than the case write-up. Whereas the case write-up is comprehensive and detailed, the oral case presentation is designed to convey information in a timely fashion that is relevant to the patient's hospitalization. The case write-up may take hours to write and fill several pages; the oral case presentation should usually be completed within five minutes.

Mistake **#40**

Not understanding the importance of the oral case presentation

The oral case presentation is the means to communicate a patient's story and clinical course to those directly responsible for developing the plan of care for that patient—often the more senior members of the primary pediatric team. In many aspects the oral case presentation is like the game "Telephone." The other members of the team only know what gets passed along to them from your presentation. Therefore, in order to make informed decisions about the appropriate diagnostic and therapeutic work-up, the entire pediatric team must be privy to an oral case presentation that is simultaneously accurate, complete, and concise. Furthermore, the oral case presentation—in an even *more* concise format—is generally utilized when asking a consulting service to evaluate one of the patients on your team.

Mistake #41

Not knowing how much time you have to present the case

Time on the floor is precious, and it is imperative that the pediatric team stays on schedule, especially during rounds. A well-presented new patient case should be complete within about five minutes, with discussion proceeding afterwards. A presentation that is shorter than this risks leaving out too many important details of the case. Presenters that go on for much longer than five minutes risk losing their audience—and thus risk not conveying essential medical information to a no longer captive audience. If it is unclear how much time you have for an oral presentation of a newly admitted patient, ask your intern or resident how much time would be reasonable to utilize for the presentation before you begin. Oral presentations of patients who were previously admitted should be much briefer.

Mistake #42

The oral case presentation has too little or too much detail

On the spectrum of too much or too little detail, medical students often tend to present patients in excessive detail when on the wards. Students often have a fear that they will leave out key details of the case if they do not present all of the data learned, or that they are too new to medicine to be the judge of what should and should not be presented to the more senior team members. These fears, while nearly universal, are ungrounded. The interns and residents are there to help out on rounds should you forget an integral component of the case. Moreover and perhaps without even realizing it, you as a medical student make decisions all the time about what to bring up and what to leave out. Just think of all that social history you acquired from that talkative patient! Don't worry if your oral presentations are a bit rough at first and don't contain all the information or contain more information than the medical team is looking for. Learning how to incorporate the pertinent positives and negatives into the oral case presentation while cutting the unimportant ones takes considerable time to master.

Success tip #39

Listen to how interns and residents give oral case presentations. By listening to others, you will hear how things are done well and not so well. Mimic the styles you think are well done and purposefully leave out aspects of other presentations you think are done poorly. Continue to draw on daily experiences to develop and refine your own style.

Mistake #43

The oral case presentation is a verbatim reading of the patient's write-up

As you probably can attest to, it's not very exciting to hear someone read the write-up out loud. The oral case presentation should maintain your listeners' attention. These five minutes should contain the telling of your patient's story to date. In this respect, the story should be well known to you; thus, you need not *read* it off of a write-up or medical record. Occasional note glancing is acceptable, especially with more medically complex patients.

Success tip #40

Have important patient information such as the patient's name, age, date of birth, medical record number, diagnosis, relevant historical information, vital signs on admission, pertinent physical examination findings, and relevant laboratory data and diagnostic studies results on a note card for quick reference.

Success tip #41

Speak clearly and confidently with enthusiasm. Don't worry that your oral case presentation is less detailed and informative than your case write-up. It's supposed to be that way. The purpose of the oral case presentation is to convey the patient's clinical scenario in the fewest words possible.

Mistake **#44**

Not practicing your oral case presentation with your resident or intern

Before giving an oral case presentation to the team, it is always good to practice your presentation with the intern or resident, or even by yourself. Practice the language and the sentence structure you will use to begin distinct aspects of the history. That way, the intern or resident can offer you suggestions on ways to improve your presentation before you give it to the entire pediatric team, including the attending. A smooth and well rehearsed medical presentation can be a pleasure to listen to, and more importantly, will engage the entire medical team in the care of your patient.

Mistake **#45**

Not seeking feedback about your oral case presentations

As with all aspects of medical education, be proactive in seeking specific feedback on your oral case presentations. Improvement comes with practice and constructive criticism.

Mistake **#46**

Not knowing how to present a patient during the oral case presentation

Listed below is a step-by-step approach to efficiently and effectively presenting a patient during the oral case presentation. Note that this approach applies to a newly admitted patient.

Step 1: Patient identification

Before presenting the patient's chief complaint, it is important to provide listeners with the full name, room number, and medical record number of the patient. As simple or obvious as this sounds, you would be surprised at how often students omit this information and begin with the chief complaint—only to be suddenly interrupted by the attending physician for the name, location, and medical record number of the patient.

Step 2: Chief complaint, reason for admission, and source of information

State the chief complaint or reason for admission. While many attending physicians prefer that the chief complaint be stated in the patient's or caregiver's own words, some prefer for the reason for admission to be the words conveyed to you by the admitting physician. Proponents of the latter approach argue that a patient's perception of the reason for admission is often not the same as that of the admitting physician and that the patient's perception, while important, is better left for the history of present illness. When conveying the chief complaint, do not forget to report its duration. It is also appropriate to mention the sources of information—mother, father, teacher, babysitter, letter from primary care physician, etc.—at this point in the presentation.

Step 3: History of present illness (HPI)

Begin the HPI with a statement that includes the patient's name, age (post-gestational age, if appropriate), ethnicity, gender, chief complaint, and *relevant* prior medical diagnoses or past medical history. An example of "relevant" would be that if the patient's chief complaint is shortness of breath, you ought to include any known history involving the respiratory tract, such as asthma or bronchopulmonary dysplasia.

After the opening statement, continue the HPI by saying, *"The patient was in his usual state of health until..."* The rest of patient's story can be presented in chronological order. In reporting the time line or chronological order of events that led up to the patient's current admission, utilize a time scale in terms of months, weeks, days, or hours prior to admission or PTA. For example, if a child has had consistent diarrhea since Tuesday and the patient is admitted on Friday, you could state, *"The patient has had persistent diarrhea since three days prior to admission."* This method, as opposed to utilizing days of the week or calendar dates, is universally accepted in the presentation of a patient's history and physical.

Symptoms should be described in detail, including onset, precipitating and palliative factors, quality and quantity, radiation and region, severity, and timing. Be sure to include all pertinent positives and negatives from the review of systems in the history of present illness. Let the differential diagnosis you are considering guide you concerning what to include.

Evaluations performed by other physicians during the course of the illness prior to hospitalization, including results of diagnostic testing as well as treatments, should be included, again at the appropriate chronological point. Since patients are generally admitted to the hospital directly after visiting their physician or the emergency room, the HPI often ends with a brief description of this visit.

Presenting the HPI	
Do...	**Don't...**
Start the HPI with an introductory statement that includes the patient's age, gender, ethnicity, relevant past medical history, and chief complaint, including duration.	Use days of the week (Monday, Tuesday etc.), but rather days prior to admission.
Present the story of the patient's illness in chronological order.	Forget to offer information about any sick contacts prior to the hospitalization.
Describe the patient's symptoms fully (onset, precipitating and palliative factors, quality, radiation and region, severity, temporal aspects).	Forget to report associated symptoms.
Include pertinent positives and negatives from the review of systems.	
Inform your listeners of how the illness has affected the patient's and family's lifestyle	
End the story with a brief description of the patient's visit to their physician or the emergency room that prompted hospital admission	

Step 4: Past medical history (PMH)

While the past medical history (PMH) in your write-up should be comprehensive (see Chapter 4), for the oral case presentation you must pass along only information that is relevant. How much information should you include? While this is largely a matter of judgment, a useful approach is to ask yourself if the information has bearing on the evaluation of the patient's current symptoms. If you determine that the information is relevant, then you should pass it along to your audience.

While the PMH can be subdivided into childhood illnesses, prior hospitalizations, and the prenatal, birth, neonatal, feeding, and growth histories, it is not necessary to provide information about each category unless the information is relevant. For example, if the prenatal, birth, and neonatal history information is not relevant to the patient's current illness, it is appropriate to say, *"the prenatal, birth, and neonatal histories are noncontributory."*

Do not repeat PMH information that you have already passed along to your audience. For example, if you discussed the patient's feeding history in the HPI, you should not repeat the feeding history when conveying the past medical history later in the presentation. You can simply state, *"the feeding history is unremarkable except as mentioned in the HPI."*

Step 5: Past surgical history (PSH)

Provide *relevant* past surgical history (PSH). If applicable, include any history of neonatal procedures such as circumcision and any associated complications such as excessive bleeding.

Presenting the PSH	
Do...	**Don't...**
Provide relevant past surgical history	Provide an extensive list of all surgical procedures performed unless they all have bearing on the patient's current illness
Provide a history of perinatal procedures and any associated complications for neonates, infants, and toddlers	

Step 6: Immunizations

Provide *pertinent* immunization history. A concise statement, *"all immunizations are up to date,"* is appropriate when applicable. Be sure to know which vaccinations have not been administered and the reasons why if the patient is not immunized fully for his or her age.

Presenting the Immunization History	
Do...	**Don't...**
Provide the relevant immunization history	Report all immunizations the patient has received unless your listeners ask you to do so
State that *"all immunizations are up to date"* if applicable to your patient	
Report any missed immunizations and the reasons why	

Step 7: Medications

Report all medications, including herbal and over-the-counter medications and supplements that the patient receives as an outpatient, as well as the indication for the medicines. When reporting the medication list, group medicines for the same condition together. Medications that you and your team started in the inpatient setting should not be reported here but rather in the assessment and plan.

Although you do not need to include the following information in your oral case presentation, know (1) the specific amount, (2) amount per kilogram, (3) amount per kilogram per dose, (4) frequency, and (5) route of each medication taken by your patient. Also inquire as to the patient's compliance with each medication. It is important to know this information to provide proper patient care. In the event that your listeners ask for any of these details, you will be able to convey the information they seek.

Presenting Medications	
Do...	**Don't...**
Report all prescription and non-prescription medications the patient is receiving	Report the indication for each medication unless asked to do so
Group medications being given for the same condition together	Report the dosage, frequency, and route of administration of each medication unless asked to do so
	Report medications that you and your team started after the patient was hospitalized

Step 8: Allergies

Discuss allergies to medications along with the reaction the patient had to the medication. For example, *"the patient has an allergy to sulfa drugs, which causes an erythematous rash."* Also include any allergies to foods, inhalants, or contacts such as poison ivy, betadine, or latex.

Step 9: Family history

Students often spend too much time conveying family history when a brief statement would suffice. While the family history section of the write-up includes an extensive list of all the diseases that have occurred in the patient's immediate and extended family, for purposes of the oral case presentation, only relevant family history should be included. If there is nothing significant to pass along from the patient's family history, it is quite reasonable to simply say, *"the family history is noncontributory."*

Step 10: Social history

The "social history" section of the write-up includes an extensive narrative of all the social interactions influencing the health and well being of the pediatric patient. In addition, it is in this section of the write-up where each individual caregiver of the patient and their responsibilities (feeding the patient, baby sitting on weeknights, taking care of the patient on weekends, etc.) are discussed in great depth. For purposes of the oral case presentation, however, only relevant social history should be included.

Presenting the Social History	
Do...	**Don't...**
Report any social history relevant to the patient's current illness	Provide a detailed social history unless it has bearing on the patient's current illness
Provide information about whom the patient lives with, and where	

Step 11: Review of systems

The "review of systems" section of the case write-up includes an extensive list of all the positive and negative ROS of each organ system. For the purposes of the oral case presentation, however, you need not be so exhaustive. Review of systems relevant to the patient's current illness should have been discussed in the HPI. Unless there is some other information that you feel is important to pass along, it will often be sufficient to say, *"The review of systems is unremarkable except as described in the HPI."* If there is additional information to pass along, you can simply say, *"Review of systems, in addition to what was already described in the HPI, include..."*

Step 12: Physical examination

Discuss the physical examination, beginning with the patient's general appearance, followed by the vital signs including, when appropriate, the percentile with respect to height, weight, head circumference (for patients less than two years of age), and BMI. The presentation of the remainder of the physical examination typically progresses from head down, by systems. Depending on the attending physician's preferences and the time allotted during rounds, the oral presentation of the physical examination may vary from a lengthy presentation including a description of every organ system, to a bullet presentation describing only abnormal findings.

If you are not sure how much to present in the physical examination, a general rule of thumb is to comment on every organ system, offering your listeners a description of relevant findings. If there are no relevant findings for a particular organ system, you may inform your audience that the examination of that particular organ system was normal. How do you decide what is relevant? A relevant finding would be any finding, either normal or abnormal, that would help your listeners determine the disease process that is accounting for the patient's symptoms or exclude other conditions in the differential diagnosis.

Presenting the Physical Examination	
Do...	**Don't...**
Begin the reporting of the physical examination with a comment about the patient's general appearance.	Forget to describe the patient's general appearance, which students commonly do.
Report the actual vital signs (temperature, pulse, respiratory rate, blood pressure).	Just say *"the patient is afebrile and the vital signs are stable."*
Follow a standard order when presenting the physical examination (from head down).	Forget to pass along orthostatic vital signs, when applicable.

Report the patient's height, weight, head circumference (for patients under two years of age), and BMI along with their percentiles.	Report the patient's head circumference unless the patient is under two years of age or there is concern for possible CNS disease.
	Make any judgments about physical examination findings. Just report the findings.
	Show ambiguity when reporting the information with comments such as *"I think I heard a murmur."*

Step 13: Laboratory data and data from chest radiographs, ECGs, and other studies

Provide the results of laboratory data, imaging studies, and other objective diagnostic tests. If your patient has abnormal laboratory test results, consider discussing the significance of these results with the intern or resident prior to presenting the data. Traditionally, laboratory data are presented with basic data first followed by more specialized results. For example:

CBC → Chemistries → Coagulation studies → Urinalysis → ECG → Radiological studies → Other laboratory data

You should know the age-appropriate normative values for the obtained data.

Presenting Test Results (Laboratory, Imaging, etc.)	
Do...	**Don't...**
Present basic data before more specialized results (see text above)	Skip around so that elements of a given laboratory test panel (CBC, Chem-10, etc.) are not given together.
Report all abnormal lab test results	Feel compelled to mention every normal test result.
Bring the ECG with you to rounds for the team to review*	Forget to bring an old ECG with you, if available, for comparison to the new ECG.
Bring any imaging studies with you to rounds for the team to review. If the study is available for viewing on the computer, bring the study onto the screen before your presentation.#	Forget to obtain or have old radiographs with you, if available, for comparison to new radiographs.
	Forget to report a normal test result if it's an important piece of information that will help your listeners exclude a condition in the differential diagnosis.

*As with vital signs and laboratory data, the ECG interval reference ranges are age-dependent and must be interpreted with the correct age-appropriate ranges in mind.

#It is a good idea to discuss the results of the imaging study with a radiologist prior to rounds so the team can be better informed of the radiologic interpretation of the film.

Step 14: Assessment/Plan

After reporting the history, physical examination, and results of laboratory and other diagnostic studies, the assessment/plan begins with a summary of the patient's clinical presentation. This summary should be brief, including important findings and data obtained from the history, physical examination, and diagnostic studies.

After the summary, discuss each of the patient's problems in descending order of importance if more than one problem exists. Problems should not be labeled by system but rather by the most specific label you can apply. For example, a patient's anemia should not be prefaced as "Heme" or even "Anemia" when a known "Microcytic Anemia" or "Iron Deficiency Anemia" is present.

For each problem, provide an assessment and a plan. In your assessment, include a prioritized differential diagnosis ranked in order of likelihood. For your working diagnosis, the diagnosis that best explains your patient's clinical presentation, explain your rationale. Discuss your reasoning and include diagnostic criteria for the working diagnosis. Support your conclusions with data, including elements of the history, physical examination, and laboratory and imaging data. Follow the assessment with an organized plan that includes other diagnostic studies to confirm your working diagnosis or exclude other conditions in the differential diagnosis. This should be immediately followed by the treatment plan.

Chapter 6

Commonly Made Mistakes On

The Daily Progress Note

You will be expected to write a daily progress note for every patient you are following on the wards. In addition, you may also be expected to write progress notes on patients followed by other students on the team, particularly on their days off. The purpose of the daily progress note is to update the reader of the patient's hospital course since the last progress note was written. Physicians, nurses, dietitians, physical therapists, and other healthcare providers rely heavily on the daily progress note, especially the assessment and plan. By quickly reviewing the progress notes, other members of the healthcare team learn not only about the patient's progress, but also about the current diagnostic and therapeutic plan as well as the patient's disposition and anticipated date of discharge. In this chapter, we will discuss commonly made mistakes on the daily progress note.

Mistake **#47**

Not reviewing how to write the progress note with the intern or resident at the beginning of the rotation

Most progress notes will use the S-O-A-P (subjective-objective-assessment-plan) format.

It is important to discuss with the intern or resident exactly what type of information should be documented in each section of the S-O-A-P progress note. While style will likely differ between members of the team, content is typically rather universal within a team and specialty.

Success tip #42

Although not officially incorporated into the S-O-A-P format, get in the habit of noting on the daily progress note the medications your patient is receiving as well as the type and route of nutrition or IV fluids your patient is receiving.

Success tip #43

If your patient is receiving antibiotics, note how many days the antibiotic has been administered. For example:

"Ceftriaxone 750 mg IV q12h (day #3)"

Success tip #44

At the end of the progress note, include a section on disposition. For example:

"Disposition (Disp): Expect patient to be discharged home tomorrow, on oral antibiotics, if patient remains afebrile and without evidence of hypoxia overnight."

Mistake #48

Not writing legibly

Physicians are notorious for poor handwriting. For whatever reason, and there *are* many, it is often easier and faster to document notes in the chart in poor penmanship. However, as a student, you will have the opportunity to put *more* time and thought into the care of *fewer* patients. Let the legibility as well as the content of your written documentation reflect that standard. It will then be more likely that those who read the patient record—including consultants who acquire history from the chart, nurses who carry out the orders in the chart, and other team members who will be assessing your ability and knowledge base—will rapidly and precisely understand your thoughts and orders. Clear and legible documentation is vital to good patient care.

Mistake #49

Not writing the date and time of the progress note

It is important to document the date and time of your patient assessment; the status of a patient can change dramatically throughout the course of the day. As an example, imagine the differing interpretation of a patient who is "difficult to arouse" when such a statement was documented in the record at 02:00 (2:00 AM) vs. 14:00 (2:00 PM). Although medical students are usually taught to date and time their notes for medical-legal purposes, the dating and timing of progress notes is also very important for proper patient care.

Success tip #45

Use 24-hour time when documenting your notes. For example, document 2:00 AM as 02:00, and 2:00 PM as 14:00.

Mistake #50

Not identifying the type of note you are writing and your educational level

The title of the note should include the type of note you are writing (e.g., progress note) and your level of medical training (e.g., MS3 for 3rd year medical student).

Mistake #51

Delaying the writing of the progress note

Generally, the intern or resident will rely on you to have the progress note completed in a timely fashion so they can co-sign your note and enter it into the permanent medical record. Don't worry if all the laboratory test results and diagnostic imaging results are not back before you complete your note; those results and their influence on the plan of care can always be added to the chart as an addendum to the progress note at a later time. Ask the more senior team members what the goal should be for completion of the daily progress note. Some will ask that you aim to have the note in the chart prior to work rounds, and others will ask for a completed note by lunch time or even later in the day. In any case, completing the daily progress note earlier rather than later will keep work from piling up later in the day and allow consultants and others who may wish to view the medical record access to a more up-to-date version of the primary team's plan of care.

Success tip #46

If the results of laboratory or diagnostic imaging tests are pending at the time you complete a progress note, indicate that in the appropriate section of the note. For example, if your patient has a microcytic anemia identified as one of their active problems and iron studies are pending, document this:

"Will follow up on this AM's iron studies, including serum iron, ferritin, and total iron binding capacity (TIBC) as those results were pending at this time."

Mistake #52

Not seeking feedback on the quality of your progress note

As with all other aspects of patient care, in order to improve your documentation skills it is important to seek feedback on your written notes from the house staff and attending physician. Effective written communication that is both concise and comprehensive is invaluable. You will master the art only with practice. There is a delicate balance between including too much and including too little in your progress note. Consult with the house staff for guidance in determining what should be recorded in your daily note.

Chapter 7

Commonly Made Mistakes During

Attending Rounds

The attending physician is the most senior member of the team. In addition to ensuring that patients assigned to the medical team receive the best possible care, the attending is also responsible for teaching the house officers and medical students on the team. Much of your interaction with the attending physician will occur during attending rounds, a period of time during which the entire team typically meets, usually in the late morning. What occurs during attending rounds may vary from day to day, particularly in relation to the team's call schedule. If your team admitted patients the day before, the team is "post-call," and the attending physician will expect to hear about these new patients during rounds. Typically, the most junior member of the team who is following the patient will present newly admitted patients to the attending physician. If there are no new patients to present, the attending physician may ask for updates on previously admitted patients, discuss interesting aspects of patients' illnesses, conduct bedside rounds, or have team members, including medical students, give talks.

Although teaching styles differ, many attending physicians like to ask students questions, especially about the disease processes their patients have. In this chapter, we will discuss commonly made mistakes during attending rounds.

Mistake #53

Not knowing your attending physician's expectations of you

Unless the attending physician has already discussed with you the precise nature of your role and responsibilities, ask the attending at the beginning of the rotation what is expected of you, particularly regarding write-ups (admission and daily progress notes) and oral case presentations. The attending physician is typically responsible for a considerable portion of your final inpatient grade, so it is important for you to know their expectations of you up front.

Mistake #54

Not knowing how to present patients to the attending

In general, there are two types of oral presentations:

- Presentations of newly admitted patients
- Presentations of established patients your attending physician is already familiar with

Mistakes that students commonly make when presenting newly admitted patients have already been discussed in detail in Chapter 5. With respect to the presentation of an established patient, simply present the patient to the attending in the same fashion that you did to the intern and resident during work rounds. (See Mistake #17: Not knowing how to efficiently present a patient during work rounds.) However, be sure to incorporate into your presentation the updated plan of care as discussed with the team earlier in the day during work rounds. The major goal when presenting established patients to the attending is to provide the attending with (1) a quick and concise update on the patient's hospital course since the previous day's rounds, and (2) the updated treatment plan and patient disposition.

Success tip #47

At the beginning of the rotation, ask the attending physician how they would like you to present your patients to them and what their specific expectations are. Then, roughly half way through the rotation, ask the attending how your performance has been and if there are any areas in which you could improve.

Mistake #55

Not having a differential diagnosis for the patient's chief complaint

The chief complaint is usually the symptom or condition that prompted the patient or the patient's family to seek medical attention. It is the job of the physician to determine the underlying cause of the symptom or condition and then formulate an adequate treatment plan. Every symptom elucidated from the patient's history usually has an extensive differential diagnosis—a list of conditions that could account for the symptom. Results from the physical examination are then used to guide the clinician in the appropriate use of laboratory investigations, diagnostic imaging, consultations, etc. to narrow the differential diagnosis to a final unifying diagnosis.

Before attending rounds, have a differential diagnosis prepared for the symptoms that led to the patient's hospitalization. When preparing your differential diagnosis, be sure to prioritize the possibilities by placing the more likely conditions causing the patient's symptoms at the top of the differential diagnosis list. Then, if you are asked for the differential, you can discuss the more likely possibilities first. This will demonstrate to the attending physician that you have used the clinical information gathered from the history and physical examination to generate a prioritized differential diagnosis from which to guide your diagnostic work-up.

In addition, when generating your differential diagnosis for the patient's symptoms, it is important to consider the life-threatening etiologies as well since these are the conditions that generally need to be excluded early in the course of the diagnostic work-up.

Success tip #48

Before attending rounds, commit to the one diagnosis that is most likely to be the cause of the patient's chief complaint, but have a list of at least 3 to 5 common and life-threatening etiologies for the patient's chief complaint as well. This way, when you are asked by the attending for your differential diagnosis, you can reply like this:

"Although there are many causes of symptom X, based on the data available at this time, I think the most probable cause is Y. However, other common and life-threatening etiologies that need to be considered are..."

Success tip #49

Familiarize yourself with the most appropriate and cost-effective work-up for the patient's presenting symptoms. For example, if the chief complaint is diarrhea, you should not only know the more common and life-threatening causes of diarrhea, but you should also be able to discuss the diagnostic work-up for diarrhea. You should be comfortable describing how you would rule in or rule out possible diagnoses through the history, physical examination, and diagnostic studies.

Mistake **#56**

Not having a differential diagnosis for a sign or physical examination finding

Just as every symptom usually has a differential diagnosis, so do signs and physical examination findings. Just as you did for the chief complaint or presenting symptoms, you will need to generate a differential diagnosis for each sign or physical examination finding— again prioritizing the possible diagnoses based on the more likely etiologies. Remember that clinical medicine is largely an exercise in problem solving. Therefore, the task of the physician is to determine whether signs and physical examination findings are related to the patient's current illness. When a finding is noted, its relevance needs to be interpreted in the context of the patient's current illness. This tenet also holds true for abnormal laboratory test results and diagnostic imaging test findings, discussed next. A step-by-step approach to interpreting findings in the context of the patient's chief complaint is discussed below.

Step-by-step approach to analyzing physical examination findings, abnormal lab test results, and imaging test findings

Step 1: Familiarize yourself with the differential diagnosis of every abnormal physical examination finding, laboratory test result, or diagnostic imaging test finding.

Step 2: Determine if the abnormal physical examination finding, laboratory test result, or diagnostic imaging test finding supports any of the conditions in your differential diagnosis.

Step 3: If the abnormal physical examination finding, laboratory test result, or diagnostic imaging test does not support any of the conditions in your differential diagnosis, consider the possibility that it is unrelated to the patient's current illness.

Step 4: If the abnormal physical examination finding, laboratory test result, or diagnostic imaging test is unrelated to the patient's current illness, develop an approach to determining its etiology.

Although an abnormal physical examination finding, laboratory test result, or diagnostic imaging test may not be directly related to the patient's current illness, it may nevertheless be important and require further evaluation.

Success tip #50

Have access to a reference book of differential diagnoses for common abnormal physical examination findings and/or an atlas of pediatric physical diagnosis.

Mistake #57

Differential diagnosis of an abnormal laboratory test result is not known

Although the history and physical examination are usually the keys to determining the diagnosis, the results of basic laboratory tests are also important adjunctive data. The results of basic laboratory tests can be very useful in determining the severity of the patient's illness, especially when the history is either unavailable or unreliable, as is often the case in pediatrics. For example, it is common for sick children to be brought to the ER by a caregiver unsure or unaware of the child's history.

Just as every symptom and sign has a differential diagnosis, so do abnormal laboratory test results. Again, it is your job not only to recognize abnormal laboratory test results, but also to interpret them in the context of the patient's current illness when prioritizing possible diagnoses; this can be done by following the step-by-step approach listed in Mistake #56.

Success tip #51

Have access to a reference book of *age-appropriate* normal values for laboratory test results. Remember, what may be a normal laboratory test result for a newborn may not be a normal laboratory test result for an adolescent, and vice versa.

Mistake **#58**

Clinical significance of an imaging test abnormality is not understood

As alluded to above, each abnormal imaging test result has its own differential diagnosis, and the job of the physician is to interpret the abnormalities in the context of the patient's current illness when prioritizing possible diagnoses. Use the step-by-step approach listed in Mistake #56 to help you elucidate the etiology of an imaging test abnormality.

Success tip #52

Have access to a reference book of *age-appropriate* normal radiographic findings as well as a reference book of abnormal radiographic findings with accompanying differential diagnoses. Again, what is a normal radiographic finding in a newborn may not be a normal radiographic finding for an adolescent, and vice versa.

Mistake **#59**

Not being well read on your patient's problems

During your clinical clerkship years, you are expected to apply the information you learned from the basic sciences towards the clinical care of your patients. As opposed to listening to lectures in the classroom, you have now advanced to more patient-centered clinical care. The focus of your education should now shift from being able to pass a test to being able to adequately care for another human being. As a clinician, you are not only responsible for yourself, but also for the well being of your patients. In order to best serve your patients, you will need to learn to integrate the information you learned from the basic sciences as well as information you obtain from independent research and apply it directly to your patient's specific problems. For your patient's problems, it should be your educational goal to know the following:

What you need to know about your patient's problems

Incidence	Laboratory studies
Epidemiology	Imaging and other
Pathogenesis	studies
Risk factors	Prognosis
Differential diagnosis	Complications
Clinical features	Therapy
(symptoms and signs)	

By knowing these features of your patient's problems, you will not only be well-prepared for questions posed by the attending, but more importantly this knowledge will positively contribute to the overall medical care of your patient.

Success tip #53

Bring an article to the team pertaining to your patient's diagnosis, should you find relevant literature. For example, both a review article on the diagnosis and treatment of pneumonia as well as an original contribution of a double-blind, randomized controlled trial (RCT) comparing two antibiotic agents for the emperical treatment of community-acquired pneumonia (CAP) would be appropriate. Accessing the medical literature will demonstrate to the team that you are independently motivated and interested, and, more importantly, will further the team's education.

Mistake #60

Not grading yourself after attending rounds

The goal is to improve your presentation skills as you progress through the pediatrics clerkship specifically, and medical school in general. After each patient presentation, ask yourself what you could do better the next time to improve on your performance. Do not hesitate to ask other members of the team—whether it be other medical students, interns, or the resident—for critical and constructive feedback.

Part II

Commonly Made Mistakes In

The Outpatient Environment

During your pediatrics outpatient clinic experience, you may be working with an individual community pediatrician or an academic pediatrician with a hospital-affiliated clinic. This time is generally spent working one-on-one with an established pediatrician. Although every physician has their own style, most will want you to see patients by yourself first. After your patient evaluation, you will generally be asked to present the patient to your preceptor, discussing the diagnostic and therapeutic implications, followed by a final visit of the patient together. Your preceptor may also request that you shadow him or her as you see patients together. You may then be allowed to see patients on your own after some time has passed and you have gained his or her trust.

Before Seeing the Patient (Outpatient Setting)

Each outpatient clinic will be slightly different in the way it's organized and run. In most offices, patients will first be checked in by the receptionist/clerk at the front desk, then have their vital signs taken by an L.V.N. or R.N., then taken to the examination room, where they then wait for the physician. Usually, it will either be your attending physician or the nurse manager who instructs you as to which patients you will be seeing in the clinic. However, in case there is any question, always be sure to check with either your attending physician or the nurse manager before seeing a patient to make sure that they are appropriate for you to interview and examine. In this chapter, we will discuss commonly made mistakes before seeing the patient in the outpatient setting.

Mistake #61

Not letting the attending physician know the patient has arrived at the clinic

Depending on the clinic, the nurses and/or clerks may notify *you* first when the patient arrives. Although it's good to take the initiative and volunteer to see the patient in a timely manner, it's best to notify the attending physician that the patient has arrived. This way, the attending can alert you to any particular information that he or she wants to elicit from the patient before you go and see the patient. Furthermore, each pediatrician has several patients in their clinic panel who are not considered "good medical student patients." Alerting the attending to who has arrived will allow them the opportunity to steer you clear of those patients.

Mistake #62

Not knowing why the patient has come to the clinic

In contrast to inpatient medicine, where all patient visits represent sick visits, in outpatient pediatrics, patient visits fall into three general categories:

● Well-child care

● Sick visits

● Follow-up visits

The routine history that you take, physical examination you perform, and anticipatory guidance you offer differ drastically across these three broad categories.

Sometimes the family doesn't even know exactly why they are in clinic, and will suggest that they are present "because they were told to be there." Through a combination of communication with the attending pediatrician, nursing and office staff, and a quick chart review, be sure to determine exactly why a patient has presented to the clinic in order to appropriately tailor their visit to that purpose.

Success tip #54

Quickly review the patient's chart prior to seeing the patient. That way, you'll be brought up to speed with the patient's problem list and the reason for this particular visit. In order to be efficient, start your chart review by examining the most recent physician/ nursing note to see what in particular, if anything, was planned for the current visit. Those patients presenting for a routine well-child visit may have a specific "well-child visit" form present in their charts.

Mistake **#63**

Not reviewing the patient's chart before seeing the patient

Failing to review the patient's chart may not only leave you in an examination room with a child and parent who are unsure of why they are there, but it may also keep you unaware of a patient with underlying chronic disease. Many parents will assume that you, as a physician or physician-in-training, already know of their child's chronic disease or other diagnoses and fail to bring this up in the conversation. It is essential that you know a patient's problem list prior to visiting with them in order to make the visit both efficient and productive.

Mistake #64

Not making a list of things to accomplish while seeing the patient

Often when you alert the attending physician as to the patient's presence, he or she will ask you to ascertain certain information during your interview with the patient. Just as you made a "scut" list of things to accomplish while you were on the wards, make a similar list of goals to accomplish while you see the patient in the outpatient setting. A similar concept applies to well-child visits. Certain questions, many of which are age-dependent, should be asked of all patients and families. Many of these are monotonous and will be forgotten if they are not available on a handy note card or piece of paper.

Success tip #55

Keep a piece of scratch paper or note card available to scribble on during the patient interview. You can then incorporate that information (and not simply forget it!) into your clinic note at the completion of the visit.

Chapter 9

Commonly Made Mistakes

While Seeing The Patient (Outpatient Setting)

Unlike the inpatient environment where you will be seeing patients and their families in either the emergency room or ward room amidst the scurry of other ongoing hospital activities, in the outpatient environment you will be seeing patients in a generally more relaxed and peaceful setting. Take this opportunity when the patient and family aren't overly anxious about being in the hospital with an acute illness to learn about the patient and his or her growth and development. In this chapter, we will discuss commonly made mistakes while seeing the patient in the outpatient setting.

Mistake **#65**

Not properly introducing yourself

The patient you are interviewing and examining expects their doctor to enter the clinic room after hearing a knock on the door. When they see a stranger (you) enter the room, the first thing they hear from you should *not* be a question about an underlying disease process or diagnosis. As a professional, you should properly introduce yourself by name, and note that you are a medical student at such-and-such university, working with Dr. X for a few days or weeks. Only then is it appropriate for you to embark on a medical interview and physical examination. As simple or obvious as this seems, you would be surprised how often eager students forget to properly identify themselves.

Mistake #66

Not taking a focused history

The history taken at a clinic visit is typically very different from the history ascertained from a patient newly admitted to the hospital. Clinic patients, while often not known to you, are very well known to the clinic (unless they are new patients), and thus do not need a thorough history taken. Rather, with established patients you should acquire an interval history, or a history dating back to their most recent previous clinic visit. However, if a patient is new to the clinic, you will be expected to elicit a complete medical history.

Success tip #56

Always determine when age-appropriate neurodevelopmental milestones were reached. This will help you get a big picture feel for how the child is developing.

Mistake #67

Not performing a complete physical examination

Even though the history taken is often a directed version, it is nonetheless important to perform a complete physical examination. Age-specific things to pay particular attention to (but certainly not the only things to examine) are listed in the following table.

Newborns	Fontanelles Red reflex Cardiac murmurs Abdominal masses Hip clicks/clunks Testicular descent (for males) Vulvar appearance (for females)
Infants	Strabismus Visual acuity Hearing acuity Tympanic membranes Leg length
Children or adolescents	Tanner stage Dental hygiene

All patients need to have their height, weight, head circumference (for those patients less than two years of age), and BMI measured. Check with the nursing staff at your clinic to determine who is responsible for each of these tasks.

Mistake #68

Not addressing the reason why the patient is at the clinic

For a variety of reasons, many of which relate to the confidence you have in your role as health care provider and the patient's parents view of you as "just a student," it can be difficult to direct the interview towards your desired goals. However, it is important that you do your best to address the actual reason that brought the child to the clinic in the first place. Learning how to best elicit the information you need in a timely and tactful fashion, that is to say, guide the conversation—without appearing overly pushy or rushed—takes time to master.

Success tip #57

If you realize that the conversation is drifting away from the goal of the visit, quickly re-direct the conversation back to the purpose of the visit in a gentle and positive manner. For example, if the purpose of a patient visit is to discuss seizure management, but all the parents want to talk about is their child's performance in soccer, consider saying something like:

"...Well, that's wonderful. Does Jimmy's great performance in soccer suggest that his seizures are being better controlled on the new medicine? I'd like to discuss with you a bit more right now about his seizure control, as we certainly wouldn't want his seizure disorder or the medicines to interfere with his soccer."

Success tip #58

At some point in your interaction with the patient and family, take a seat on anything available in the examination room—whether it be the examination bench itself, a stool, chair, whatever—even if just for a few moments. Being seated will give the appearance that you are relaxed and at ease with the family, and that you have the time to take a seat and personally interact with the patient and the patient's family.

Mistake #69

Not listening to the parents

Although each clinic visit usually has a preset purpose, it is important to pay attention to what concerns the parents express, as these will be where their focus lies. Oftentimes, it is not until the end of the interview that the parents will state their worries regarding their child. For example, at the end of the interview as you are walking towards the door, a parent may state *"Oh, and doctor, it's OK if my child is eating more, drinking more, and urinating more at his age, right?"* Remember, parents want what's best for their child, and they often are the first to notice that something is wrong with their child, typically well before a health professional would! Take parents seriously when they express genuine concern.

Mistake #70

Not asking the patient and parents if there are any concerns in addition to the chief complaint or reason for clinic visit

Always ask your patient and his or her family members when they are present if there are any additional questions or concerns that they would like to discuss before you conclude the visit. Even if you know that the attending physician will be back in the examination room in just a few moments, this is an excellent habit to get yourself into. You will be surprised how many things of import emerge after this question is posed.

Mistake #71

Not observing the patient's interaction with the caregiver

A lot of information can be obtained simply by observing how the pediatric patient interacts with the caregiver. An astute and experienced clinician can usually tell when there is tension between the child and one or more of the caregivers or family members. This may be the lone finding that leads to the discovery of child neglect or abuse.

Success tip #59

As you walk into the room, pause for a moment and observe the interaction between the patient and caregivers. Particularly with infants, note if the infant goes towards the caregiver for comfort when approached by a strange person—you! If you sense tension or notice an unusual interaction, notify the attending physician of your observations, as this could be a red flag that something more serious is occurring in the home environment.

Mistake **#72**

Not observing the patient for their display of neuro-developmental milestones

Much of pediatrics is focused on growth and development, and a plethora of information can be obtained simply by watching the child in his or her environment.

Success tip #60

Review age-appropriate neurodevelopmental milestones with the patient's age in mind prior to examining a patient so you can accurately gauge whether or not the child is developing at an age-appropriate level.

Mistake **#73**

Not asking the patient and parents if they have any questions before you leave the room

As noted above, this is a question that should be asked of all parents. If you cannot appropriately answer a parent's question or if the family raises a new concern, be sure to bring it up with the attending pediatrician.

Success tip #61

Conclude each visit with a phrase such as the following:

"Is there anything else I can do for you or answer for you before I go?"

Chapter 10

Commonly Made Mistakes

When Presenting the Patient (Outpatient Setting)

In the inpatient environment, you will usually be presenting patients in front of the entire medical team— the other medical students, interns, resident, and attending physician. In the outpatient environment it is often just you and the attending discussing the patient. Although the outpatient setting is usually more relaxed, the content of the patient presentation should nonetheless be complete. You should take advantage of the more personal interaction you will have with your attending physician in the outpatient setting to learn about his or her philosophy and approach to medicine. In this chapter, wte will discuss commonly made mistakes when presenting the patient in the outpatient setting.

Mistake **#74**

Not understanding the importance of the oral case presentation

As mentioned previously, it is essential that you develop proficiency in the oral case presentation. Clearly and concisely conveying the pertinent positives and negatives of a patient's history and physical examination is one of those key skills that is essential to the practice of good medicine. Many students focus their efforts—especially in the outpatient clinic setting—on extensively documenting the patient visit in the chart, failing to spend a few moments pre-planning the oral presentation in one's head. While such thorough written documentation may be helpful during a subsequent patient visit, it does little to help in the diagnostic and therapeutic process at the moment. Make an active choice to concentrate much of your efforts in thinking about the diagnostic dilemma at hand rather than side-stepping the thinking by focusing on documentation of the patient presentation. This will truly *help* your patient.

Mistake #75

Not knowing how to present clinic patients

A step-by-step approach to presenting the outpatient to your preceptor follows.

How to present a patient in the outpatient clinic

Step 1: State the patient's name, age (post-gestational age, if appropriate), ethnicity, and gender. Also, if appropriate, state the patient's percentile with respect to height, weight, head circumference, and body mass index (BMI).

Step 2: State the last time the patient was seen at the clinic if the patient is a return patient. If the patient is a new patient, make sure the attending knows that the patient has never been seen in the clinic before.

Step 3: State the chief complaint or reason for the clinic visit. Noting that this appointment is for a routine well-child examination is appropriate.

Step 4: State the history of present illness (HPI) in chronological order. If the patient is being seen for a sick visit, focus the HPI on the pertinent positives and negatives relevant to the chief complaint. If the patient is being seen for a well child visit, focus the HPI on acquired milestones or any significant events or interval illnesses in the patient's life since the last clinic visit. If the patient is living with a chronic disease, give an interval history on the status of the underlying disease.

Step 5: For a sick visit, provide any pertinent past medical history relevant to the chief complaint.

Step 6: Provide the immunization history.

Step 7: List all medications the patient is receiving, including all herbal or over-the-counter medications or supplements. Note the specific amount, amount per kilogram, amount per kilogram per dose, frequency, and route.

Step 8: List allergies to medications along with the specific reaction observed. For example, *"Allergy to sulfa drugs, which causes an erythematous rash."*

Step 9: Provide the social history, including the child's caretakers. This section should not receive much attention if the patient is well known to the clinic attending and there have not been any significant alterations in the social history since the previous visit. Note whether or not the child attends school or day care.

Step 10: For a sick visit, provide any family history relevant to the chief complaint.

Step 11: Provide the complete review of systems (ROS). Inquire about how the child is eating, voiding (urination and stooling), and whether or not the child has lost or gained any weight. If the child has presented for a sick visit, much of this data may have already been presented in the HPI and need not be repeated here. You should supply information regarding how the child is progressing along his or her growth curves with respect to height, weight, head circumference (for those patients less than two years of age), and BMI.

Step 12: Provide the physical examination. Start with general appearance and vital signs. You should perform a complete physical examination. Only if you are directed to do so by the attending physician is it acceptable in the clinic setting to perform a focused physical examination based on the patient's chief complaint. For example, if the patient's chief complaint is ear pain and fever, you may not need to spend time performing a complete neurological examination. You would, however, need to perform a comprehensive HEENT examination in addition to examining the cardiovascular and respiratory systems, the abdomen, and other pertinent organ systems.

Step 13: Provide additional data that is important and available, including laboratory results and the findings of other diagnostic procedures such as diagnostic imaging, ECG, echocardiogram, etc. Such data will typically be available only in follow-up cases. The acute or new patient will generally not yet have laboratory data available in the clinic.

Step 14: Give the assessment and plan. Begin with a concise summary of the patient and his or her problems. Next, prioritize the patient's clinical problems. For each new problem, formulate a differential diagnosis ranked in order of likelihood. Finally, discuss a clinical plan of care to address each problem.

Mistake #76

Not seeking feedback about your oral case presentations

Just like in the inpatient setting, you should be proactive about seeking feedback on your oral case presentations in the outpatient setting. As stated above, improvement only comes with practice and constructive criticism. Don't be offended by criticism; rather, use the comments and suggestions you receive to improve the quality of your presentations.

Success tip #62

Depending on the way the clinic operates, you may discuss the patient's case with the attending physically in the patient's room in the presence of a nurse or other ancillary staff member as they are preparing to give vaccinations, entertaining the child, etc. If this is the case, seek feedback from those individuals as well.

Chapter 11

Commonly Made Mistakes

When Completing Clinic Paperwork (Outpatient Setting)

In most cases, more paperwork has to be completed per patient visit in the outpatient setting than in the inpatient setting. After the initial H&P (history and physical) in the inpatient environment, usually only a single progress note is written each day for each hospitalized patient. For each outpatient clinic visit, however, each patient often needs to have a progress note, standardized forms such as TB questionn aires, neurodevelopmental milestone acquisition forms, and school performance checklists, as well as a billing sheet completed before the end of the visit. This is not to mention that in a typical clinic day the attending physician may be seeing twenty to thirty patients! Thus, timely and accurate completion of clinic paperwork is essential to the survival of the clinic and efficient patient care. In this chapter, we will discuss commonly made mistakes when completing clinic paperwork in the outpatient setting.

Mistake **#77**

Not inquiring as to who is responsible for the clinic note

In the majority of clinic settings, the medical student will be expected to document their patient interaction in the traditional S-O-A-P format. The attending will typically read this note and then add comments—including an abbreviated assessment and plan. In some clinics, typically in the private practice setting, attending physicians will write their own complete clinic notes, occasionally even asking students not to leave documentation in the chart. Be sure to check with your preceptor before leaving written notes in the chart.

Mistake #78

Not completing the clinic note in a timely manner

During your inpatient rotation your intern or resident relies on you to have the progress note completed in a timely fashion. In the clinic your preceptor also relies on you to keep up with the paperwork, especially if you are responsible for the clinic note. By completing your clinic notes in a timely fashion, you and your preceptor won't have to stay too long after clinic has ended to finish the necessary documentation.

Success tip #63

If possible, complete your clinic note before staffing the patient with your preceptor. That way, after you and the attending discuss the patient, the attending can quickly amend your note if needed, adding his or her comments. This will prevent you and your preceptor from having to stay too long after clinic has ended writing and reviewing notes.

Mistake **#79**

Not having the attending physician co-sign your clinic note before it is entered into the medical record

For legal and billing purposes, it is necessary to have the attending physician on record co-sign your notes before they are entered into the medical record. In a busy clinic, the attending physician will often be moving quickly from patient to patient in order to see everyone. As alluded to above, having your clinic note completed before staffing your patient with the attending will facilitate the flow of patient traffic. However, in a rush to move on to the next patient, the attending may forget to sign the note; if this happens, remind the attending of the need for their signature.

Mistake **#80**

Not inquiring as to who is responsible for the billing sheet

In most outpatient clinics, the billing sheet will be attached to the patient's chart and will need to be completed before the patient leaves the office. While most of the actual medical coding will probably be done by ancillary personnel, the physician is usually responsible for documenting the patient's diagnoses that were relevant to the clinic visit. For accurate reporting and billing, each diagnosis listed on the billing sheet should be documented and addressed in the clinic note. It is beneficial to your future employment as a physician to familiarize yourself with the fundamentals of medical billing as a student. Volunteer to complete the physician sections of the billing sheet.

Success tip #64

Familiarize yourself with the different types of medical codes used for billing purposes, including ICD (international classification of diseases), DRG (diagnosis related group), CPT (common procedural terminology), and HCPCS (HCFA [health care financing administration] common procedural coding system).

Mistake **#81**

Not notifying the attending physician before leaving the clinic

Always touch base with the attending physician prior to leaving the clinic. That way, teaching points not already made throughout the clinic day can be addressed, and any questions that you may have regarding the care of the patients you saw can be asked. The outpatient care of patients often differs significantly from their inpatient care. While most of medical school is based on the hospital-based inpatient model of patient care, it is important to familiarize yourself with how an outpatient facility operates, since it is in the outpatient setting that most physicians spend the majority of their clinical careers.

Part III

Commonly Made Mistakes In

The Nursery

Statistically speaking, the single day in each person's life that is associated with the highest degree of morbidity and mortality is day-of-life one (the day of birth). Neonatology, thus, is a unique field in medicine in general and in pediatrics specifically. Those who specialize in neonatology seek to care for the youngest and smallest patients, consistently allowing pre-term neonates of younger and younger gestational ages to survive from what was considered a pre-viable age just a few years ago. Most of the interaction medical students have with neonates is in the Level I nursery, or normal newborn (well baby) nursery. In this setting, newborns are typically term or near-term, healthy and happy, occasionally struggling through the transition from fetal life to extra-placental life with the need for short-term supplemental oxygen or requiring phototherapy for hyperbilirubinemia. Depending on the medical school, students in some cases may also have the opportunity to help care for critically ill neonates. In any event, you will quickly come to see that truly caring for a newborn baby involves caring for the neonate's family as well. These can be extremely challenging yet rewarding experiences.

To better acclimate you to the world of neonatology, we list below a sampling of terms and their definitions that will be useful to know:

PART III
THE NURSERY

Term	Definition
Preterm	Less than 37 weeks gestation
Term	37 to 41 6/7 weeks gestation
Postterm	42 weeks gestation or more
Macrosomia	4000 grams or greater birth weight
NBW	Normal birth weight, 2500 to 3999 grams
LBW	Low birth weight, 1500 to 2499 grams
VLBW	Very low birth weight, 1000 to 1499 grams
ELBW	Extremely low birth weight. Less than 1000 grams
AGA	Appropriate for gestational age based on weight, length, and FOC (frontal-occipital circumference)
LGA	Large for gestational age based on weight, length, and FOC (frontal-occipital circumference)
SGA	Small for gestational age based on weight, length, and FOC (frontal-occipital circumference)
IUGR	Intrauterine growth retardation
GIR	Glucose infusion rate
Level I nursery	Normal newborn nursery
Level II nursery	High-risk nursery
Level III nursery	Neonatal intensive care unit (NICU)

Chapter 12

Commonly Made Mistakes During

Prerounds (Nursery)

In Chapter 1 we discussed mistakes that students make during pediatric prerounds. In general, prerounds on neonates are similar to prerounds on other pediatric patients in the hospital and, as such, the mistakes discussed in Chapter 1 are certainly relevant to prerounds performed in the nursery as well. The focus of this chapter is on common mistakes students make during prerounds in the nursery.

Mistake #82

Not checking with the nurse before examining the patient

Neonatology nurses try hard to maintain feeding schedules and sleep-wake cycles for the babies. This is especially true in the NICU (neonatal ICU), where the nursing staff works to create as normal an environment as possible for the many neonates that live there for the first several weeks, even months, of their lives. Check with the baby's nurse in the NICU or nursery or the mother's nurse if the baby is on the maternity wards before unbundling or waking up a baby for an examination. The nurse will appreciate this professional courtesy.

Success tip #65

Try to examine the patient every day at a pre-designated time set by you and the nurses, based on the patient's feeding schedule and sleeping schedule. Examining a newborn either just prior to or immediately after feeding typically works best.

Success tip #66

If the mother is feeding the patient, either by breast or bottle, wait until the feeding session is completed before asking to examine the infant. This will prevent the mother from feeling hurried to complete the feeding session—which is of paramount importance for the infant.

Mistake **#83**

Not discussing the care of the patient with the family

A new baby is the most precious gift a family can have. Families typically want to spend every possible moment with their new family member. In the hospital, however, the family must contend with nurses, social workers, doctors, and medical students who also need to spend time with the child in order to complete a number of distinct tasks aimed at ensuring the health and proper care of the newborn. While true in the healthy baby, what is especially true in the sick child is that the medical team will want to spend more time with, perform more diagnostic procedures and blood draws on, and initiate more therapeutic interventions for the neonate. This is undoubtedly very scary for parents. In an attempt to reduce such fears and make the hospital environment as comfortable as possible, make it a point to brief the family daily regarding the status of their baby. Update them on the results of any newly obtained diagnostic tests or studies and discuss with them the reasons for, and implications of, any therapeutic interventions currently being utilized, including antibiotics or other medicines, UV lights, or IV fluids. In short, involve them in the care of their own child. Should the family have questions that you can't answer or do not feel comfortable answering, tell them that you will discuss their questions with the rest of the medical team during rounds and that you or another member of the team will return with the information they seek.

Success tip #67

Touch base—personally if possible, or by telephone—with the patient's family at least once a day to inform them of the status of their baby.

Mistake #84

Not checking for results of laboratory or other diagnostic tests of mother and baby

Typically, the mother has her blood drawn for the prenatal screen prior to delivery, although occasionally this is not done until labor begins. The prenatal screen consists of a number of diagnostic tests and antibody titers including the blood type, Rh antibody status, HBsAb, HBsAg, HIV, RPR, and Rubella. In addition, many obstetricians document the Group B Streptococcus (GBS) status of the mother via a urine screen or vaginal or rectal swab, as GBS vaginal colonization is associated with an increased risk of neonatal GBS sepsis. If not already documented in the newborn's chart, the results of these tests should be determined and documented in the medical record as they will influence the medical care of the neonate. For example, it is extremely important to know if the mother is HIV positive or Hepatitis B surface antigen positive so that the baby can receive timely intervention and therapy. Usual blood work performed on the baby at the time of birth will include a blood type and Rh status,which are determined from cord blood and *not* with an additional blood draw from the baby. Other blood work drawn at birth for high-risk infants include a CBC with differential when concerned about neonatal sepsis, or a Coombs test when concerned about possible Rh isoimmunization. Capillary blood glucose levels are determined via dextrose sticks in infants at high risk for hypoglycemia (neonates born to diabetic mothers), or who are demonstrating symptoms consistent with that diagnosis. Chemistries and bilirubin levels are sent when appropriate.

Success tip #68

Always attempt to review the mother's chart, as the results of her prenatal studies (serum, ultrasound results, etc.) are often located in the obstetrics records. It is here that you will also find documentation of pre-birth perinatal complications, such as premature rupture of membranes (PROM), prolonged maternal fever, non-reassuring fetal heart tracing, and others.

Mistake **#85**

Not knowing normative data values for the neonate

As discussed previously, normal values for neonates with respect to vital signs, laboratory values, nutritional caloric requirements, etc. may not be normal values for other ages of pediatric patients. You will need to know what the normative values are for the neonate in order to interpret the data you obtain during prerounds on the newborn child.

Success tip #69

Have access to a reference book containing the
normative values for the neonate with respect to vital
signs, laboratory values, radiographic findings, and
nutritional caloric requirements.

Chapter 13

Commonly Made Mistakes During

Work Rounds (Nursery)

In Chapter 2, we discussed commonly made mistakes during pediatric work rounds. Nursery work rounds are similar to pediatric ward work rounds and, as such, the mistakes discussed in Chapter 2 are certainly relevant to nursery work rounds as well. The focus of this chapter is on common mistakes students make during work rounds that are particular to the nursery.

Mistake **#86**

Not knowing how to present a neonate on work rounds

Presenting a neonate on work rounds is somewhat different from presenting other pediatric patients. (See Mistake #17: Not knowing how to efficiently present a patient during work rounds.) Presentation style and content differ in many significant aspects. Following is a detailed, step-by-step approach to efficiently presenting a neonate during work rounds.

Step-by-step approach to the pediatrics work rounds presentation (nursery)

Step 1: Present the patient to the team by giving the patient's name, age in terms of day of life (e.g., DOL #2), post-gestational age, ethnicity, gender, pregnancy and/or perinatal complications if present, and any pertinent maternal studies. In essence, this birth history takes the place of the traditional HPI for older patients.

Example: Michael Cruz is a term LGA, 38 4/7 week post-gestational age Hispanic male, on day of life #2, born via normal spontaneous vaginal delivery to a 27 year-old G_2 $P_{1\to2}$ mother with a pregnancy complicated by the development of gestational (diet-controlled) diabetes in the third trimester. The patient is currently in the Level II nursery secondary to the finding of increased work of breathing at delivery and persistent post-natal hypoglycemia. Spontaneous rupture of membranes occurred 4 hours prior to delivery with clear fluid, the mother was and remains afebrile, and her Group B Strep status is negative.

Step 2: Present the subjective data, which should include the patient's current status as well as any events or complications that have occurred or developed since the previous day's rounds.

Example: No new events occurred overnight. The nurses report that the patient did not have any episodes of apnea or bradycardia; they also report that he fed well— both breast and bottle feeding at the present time—and did not report any episodes of jitteriness or fussiness. There were no hypoglycemic episodes noted overnight, although the patient does continue to receive IV dextrose with D12.5W + NaCl 2 mEq/100mL + KCl 2 mEq/100mL at a glucose infusion rate (GIR) of 8 mg/kg/min.

Step 3: Present the objective data, beginning with the vital signs.

Example: Over the past 24 hours, the T_{max} was 98.8°F, with T_C of 98.6°F. Current pulse is 130, respiratory rate 45, blood pressure 75/40, and O_2 saturation 97% on room air. The weight today is 4200 grams—a decrease of 85 grams from yesterday and roughly 2% below the *patient's birth weight of 4285 grams. Ins were 90 mL/kg/ day via IV fluids with D12.5W + NaCl 2 mEq/100mL + KCl 2 mEq/100mL at a glucose infusion rate (GIR) of 8 mg/kg/min plus breastfeeding PO ad lib; urinary output was 302 mL's or ~3 mL/kg/hour, and the patient had 2 stools.*

Step 4: Present the physical examination findings from your most recent examination. (See Appendix F for a discussion of the normal newborn examination.) For newborns, make sure to assess the following:

- **The cranium.** A bulging or sunken fontanelle is abnormal. Overriding sutures might suggest trauma to the head during labor, and a cephalohematoma may promote worsening hyperbilirubinemia.

- **The respiratory system.** Grunting, nasal flaring, or retractions are consider pathologic.

- **The cardiovascular system.** Assess for the presence of adequate peripheral perfusion and identify any cardiac murmurs present. Most newborns will have the audible murmur of a closing ductus arteriosus at some point, and it just may be that you are listening at the time!   Other murmurs may present early, as well.

- **The gastrointestinal system.** A distended abdomen may present in a number of pathologic conditions, but may also occur in those babies receiving CPAP. Be sure to listen for the presence of bowel sounds.

- **Skin color.** Assess for evidence of proper perfusion; cyanosis is OK when peripheral (termed acrocyanosis), but pathologic if central, on the mouth, lips, or nose.

- **The musculoskeletal system.** Assess for evidence of a broken clavicle, which may occur during the birthing process, or congenital hip dysplasia, suggested by the presence of a hip click/clunk.

Present both pertinent positives and pertinent negatives from the physical examination.

Example: Physical examination is notable for a soft and flat anterior fontanelle, clear breath sounds with good air exchange, no cardiac murmur, bowel sounds with no evidence of abdominal distension, and extremities that are warm, pink, and well-perfused.

Step 5: Present any new laboratory test results. Old results may be presented if needed as a reference point. Also state any pertinent interventions being performed that may influence the laboratory test results.

Example: The patient's peripheral glucose level this morning was 124 mg/dl, and over the past 24 hours his glucose levels have been 102 mg/dl, 88 mg/dl, 90 mg/dl, and 86 mg/dl by dextrose-stick measured every 6 hours. Of note, the patient's glucose level at 2 hours of life was 35 mg/dl prior to any intervention. He is currently breastfeeding PO ad lib and receiving D12.5W + NaCl 2 mEq/100mL + KCl 2 mEq/100mL at a glucose infusion rate (GIR) of 8 mg/kg/min.

Step 6: If applicable, present the results of any diagnostic studies or imaging test.

Example: A chest radiograph obtained yesterday revealed no infiltrates, effusions, or cardiomegaly. However, there was fluid noted in the major fissures bilaterally.

Step 7: Discuss the problems and treatment plan. The problems should be discussed in order of decreasing importance. Provide an assessment for each problem followed by the management plan.

Example: Problem #1 is increased work of breathing at delivery. Although the patient is at risk for respiratory pathology secondary to being an infant of a diabetic mother, his clinical examination is now without evidence of respiratory pathology and his chest radiograph findings are more consistent with a diagnosis of transient tachypnea of the newborn (TTN—also sometimes called 'retained fetal lung fluid') than with the respiratory distress syndrome (RDS). His room air oxygen saturation is 97% and he is breathing comfortably, again arguing for a diagnosis of resolving TTN. At the present time, he requires no intervention with regards to his respiratory status, and we will continue to monitor him clinically.

Problem #2 is persistent hypoglycemia after birth. As with many children born to diabetic mothers, this patient is at risk for persistent post-natal hypoglycemia secondary to hyperinsulinism. This morning, his glucose level was 124 mg/dl with a glucose infusion rate of 8 mg/kg/min plus breastfeeding PO ad lib, and his glucose levels have been above 80 mg/dl for the past 24 hours. The plan will be to decrease his glucose infusion rate (GIR) to 6 mg/kg/min and monitor his glucose levels every 6 hours. If the glucose remains stable for two to three subsequent dextrose sticks, we will likely reduce the GIR by an additional 2 mg/kg/min to 4 mg/kg/min, and continue to monitor glucose levels.

Chapter 14

Commonly Made Mistakes While

On Call (Nursery)

In Chapter 3, we discussed commonly made mistakes while on call. In general, being on call in the nursery is similar to being on call on the general pediatric ward and, as such, the mistakes discussed in Chapter 3 are certainly relevant for nursery call as well. The focus of this chapter is on common mistakes students make while on call in the nursery.

Mistake #87

Not knowing where the Labor and Delivery (L&D) suites are located

Although clerkships differ significantly by hospital and institution, many nursery experiences will include the newborn assessment and resuscitation, in the delivery room, as a required part of the rotation. If this is the case at your school, be sure to locate the labor and delivery (L&D) suites prior to being on call. It's very difficult to assist in the assessment and/or resuscitation of a newborn if you can't locate the birthing room or operating room where the delivery is being performed! In an urgent case, the intern or resident will not have time to page you or find you, to direct you to the proper place.

Mistake #88

Not knowing the approach to evaluating and assessing a newborn

Below we have listed questions that you should ask yourself when evaluating and assessing a newborn. (Refer to Appendix F for information about the normal newborn examination.)

When evaluating and assessing a neonate, ask yourself the following questions:

- What is the estimated gestational age of the baby?

- How was the baby delivered? (Normal spontaneous vaginal delivery, forceps- or vacuum-assisted vaginal delivery, cesarean section)

- If the baby wasn't delivered vaginally, why not? Possible reasons: failure to progress, fetal distress, breech position, etc.

- Was there meconium present at birth or at the rupture of membranes?

- Did the membranes rupture spontaneously or were they ruptured by the obstetrician?

- How long were the membranes ruptured prior to delivery?

- Was the baby breathing or crying at delivery?

- Did the baby have good muscle tone at delivery?

- Was the baby pink at delivery? If the baby was blue, where was he or she blue—centrally or peripherally?

- Was there any need for resuscitation of the neonate at delivery? Resuscitation includes the requirement for any medical intervention, such as the delivery of artificial breaths or oxygen, intubation, medicines, etc.

- Were there any abnormal maternal studies known prior to delivery?

- What is the mother's Group B Strep status? If necessary, did the mother receive appropriate intrapartum antibiotic prophylaxis?

- Did the mother have a fever?

- What were the APGAR scores at 1 and 5 minutes?

Mistake #89

Not writing admission orders for the babies you admit

The admission orders for neonates are slightly different than the typical admission orders for other pediatric patients (see Mistake #32: Relying on your intern or resident to write the patient's admission orders); however, it is beneficial for your education to become proficient in writing admission orders for neonates.

Success tip #70

Use the mnemonic ADC VAAN DIMLS to aid in writing your admission orders. See table below.

Writing admission orders in the nursery		
Component of admission order	**Write...**	**Example**
Admit to	Ward team Attending physician (include pager number) Resident (include pager number) Intern (include pager number)	*Admit to Level II nursery; Attending—Dr. Jones (beeper 1122); Resident— Dr. Clark (beeper 3344); Intern—Dr. Williams (beeper 5566).*
Diagnosis	The condition/diagnosis that the patient is being admitted for, if known. It is also acceptable to place a symptom such as increased work of breathing.	*Diagnosis—increased work of breathing; hypoglycemia. An alternative diagnosis, but still acceptable, is "normal newborn."*
Condition	Good/stable/fair/poor/ guarded	*Condition—stable.*
Vital signs	Per routine or q shift is usually sufficient for healthy newborns in the nursery.	*Vital signs—per routine.*
Activity	Incubator, warmer, or open crib	*Activity—open crib.*
Allergies	List drug allergies here. Most newborn initially will have "no known drug allergies" noted. (Of note, use latex-free material when handling neonates born with spina bifida occulta.)	*Allergies—NKDA.*

Nursing	Instructions for nursing should be placed here. These may include contact precautions for infectious particles, strict I/O's, neuro-checks, fingerstick glucose measurements, nasogastic suctioning, checking feeding residuals, call intern or resident if…, etc.	*Nursing—strict I/O's, daily weights, strict hand washing after interacting with patient. Notify house officer for temperature > 100.4°F. Finger-stick glucose levels q6h; notify house officer for glucose level < 45 mg/dl.*
Diet	NPO/breastfeed/formula (specify which type)/clear liquids/refeeding diet/regular diet. In neonates, you will need to specify the volume, frequency, and route of administration of the food item.	*Diet—breastfeed PO ad lib if respiratory rate < 60/min.*
IV fluids	Order the type and amount of IV fluids you want the patient to receive. Fluid should be ordered as a rate per unit time (typically mL's/hr).	*IV fluids—D12.5W + NaCl 2 mEq/100 mL + KCl 2 mEq/100 mL at 16 mL/hr, which equals a glucose infusion rate of 8 mg/kg/min (based on the patient's birth weight of 4285 grams).*
Medications	Specify the medication as well as the total dosage, dosage per kilogram, frequency, route of administration, and indication if the medication is given on a prn basis. For instance, if the child weighs 8 kg and you want to prescribe Ampicillin, write Ampicillin 800mg (=100 mg/kg/dose) IV q6h.	*Medications— Acetaminophen 60 mg (~15 mg/kg/dose) PO q6h prn temperature > 100.4°F.*

Labs	Specify when and what type of laboratory tests should be ordered.	*Labs—Chem-7 and bilirubin in AM.*
Special	Include anything else here that you haven't listed above, including any non-laboratory studies that need to be performed. All radiological studies should have a separate requisition form, which includes the type of study to be performed, indication for the study, and essential patient history, filled out in advance.	*Special—Chest radiograph (PA and lateral) in AM to evaluate increased work of breathing. Requisition form in chart.*

Mistake #90

Not notifying your resident when the baby is seriously ill or has had a change in their clinical course

It is *extremely* important for you to notify the intern and/or resident *immediately* when the clinical status of your neonatal patients changes. Newborns can get sick and decompensate *very* quickly, so timely intervention is of essence to proper medical care. Neonates have very little reserve and very immature organs, so they do not respond to stress and illness the same way an older child would. Expect changes and be prepared for prompt intervention; then, hopefully, your neonatal patients will develop appropriately.

Chapter 15

Commonly Made Mistakes On

Write-Ups (Nursery)

In general, write-ups for newborn patients are similar to write-ups for standard pediatric patients (see Chapter 4); however, differences do exist. Commonly made mistakes on the neonatal write-up are discussed below.

Mistake **#91**

Not knowing what to include in the neonatal write-up

The write-up for a neonate is slightly different than the write-up for other pediatric patients (see Mistake #39: Not knowing what to include in the write-up). The content of the write-up is usually divided among the elements listed in the following box.

Elements of the neonatal write-up

Patient identification
Method of delivery
Perinatal events
Maternal obstetrical history
Prenatal history
Family history
Physical examination
Laboratory data / other studies
Assessment
Plan

Unlike the more standardized format of the traditional pediatric case write-up, the expected content of the neonatal write-up often varies by institution. Review with your attending physician his or her expectations for the neonatal case write-up.

Mistake #92

Not adequately addressing the maternal obstetrical and prenatal history

In assessing the newborn and anticipating potential perinatal complications, it is crucial to know and document the entire maternal obstetrical history. For example, it is helpful to know at what age the mother became pregnant with the child, whether or not she received prenatal care and if so, whether the care was routine or infrequent, whether she exposed the fetus to alcohol, tobacco, or illicit substances during the pregnancy, whether she had any pre-pregnancy health issues (such as diabetes or heart disease), whether she had any pregnancy-related complications (such as hypertension or gestational diabetes), and whether she has had previous children and whether or not she had complications with those pregnancies. If the mother has had previous pregnancies, determine whether those prior pregnancies took place with the same father as in the present gestation. For sick newborns, it is especially important to obtain reports from any studies performed during the pregnancy—particularly ultrasound reports. Amniocentesis results, triple screen data, and other fetal studies should be retrieved as well.

Success tip #71

If possible, in addition to a thorough chart review, take an obstetrical history directly from the mother. Although this is traditionally the job of the obstetrics team, it can never hurt to obtain the appropriate information from the primary source yourself. You will experience numerous instances where important history is missed and key questions relevant to the health of the baby are not asked by the obstetrics service.

Mistake **#93**

Not documenting the prenatal labs or birth labs

As discussed above, the traditional prenatal labs usually include a number of diagnostic tests and antibody titers including blood type, Rh antibody status, HBsAb, HBsAg, HIV, RPR, Rubella, and GBS status. Laboratory values obtained on the neonate at birth are typically determined from cord blood and *not* from a separate blood draw from the baby, and usually consist of a blood type and Rh antibody status. Other blood tests done at birth for high-risk infants include a CBC with differential when there is concern about neonatal sepsis, and a Coombs test when there is concern about hemolysis. Capillary blood glucose levels are determined via dextrose sticks in infants at high-risk for hypoglycemia, such as neonates born to diabetic mothers, or infants who are demonstrating symptoms consistent with that diagnosis. Other chemistries, bilirubin levels, and liver function tests (LFTs) are sent when appropriate. The results of these tests all have implications for the health of the neonate, and thus should be documented in your write-up.

Mistake #94

Not calculating the gestational age of the neonate by clinical examination

Although most obstetricians and mothers have a good estimate of what gestational age the baby is, remember that it is just that—an estimate. The estimate was most likely obtained from the mother's history of her LMP along with data obtained from an early ultrasound; however, those patients who are considered "poor historians," had sparse to no prenatal care, and/or failed to have an early ultrasound performed, will have an estimated gestational age that may be over four weeks off from the actual date. Use the Ballard score obtained from your physical examination to calculate the baby's gestational age. If the Ballard score derived-date differs from the OB estimated-date by more than a couple of weeks, treat the baby as if he or she is the gestational age determined by the Ballard score.

Chapter 16

Commonly Made Mistakes On

The Oral Case Presentation (Nursery)

In general, the oral case presentation for newborn patients is similar to the oral case presentation for standard pediatric patients (see Chapter 5); however, differences do exist. Commonly made mistakes on the neonatal oral case presentation are discussed below.

Mistake #95

Not knowing how to present a neonate during the oral case presentation

The oral case presentation of a neonate is slightly different than the oral case presentation of other pediatric patients. (See Mistake #46: Not knowing how to present a patient during the oral case presentation.) Below is a step-by-step approach to an efficient neonatal oral case presentation.

Step-by-step approach to the neonatal oral case presentation

Step 1: Introduce the patient by stating the name and post-gestational age, ethnicity, and gender. The age should be given in terms of day of life, for example, DOL #2.

Step 2: Note the method of delivery and discuss any relevant perinatal complications. If the patient requires Level II or Level III nursery care, note the reason.

Step 3: State significant perinatal events and maternal history, including single episodes or chronic conditions of complications that presented during the pregnancy. Include in this section the prenatal screen laboratory results, maternal Group B Streptococcus status, and the results of other important diagnostic laboratory examinations performed on the mother or fetus prior to delivery.

Step 4: Provide a brief family history, noting in particular a family history of genetic disorders, metabolic disorders, or perinatal complications. Be sure to inquire as to the outcome of previous pregnancies, especially when there is a discrepancy between the number of gestations and the number of live children and, if so, distinguish between prior spontaneous and elective abortions.

Step 5: Provide the physical examination:

- Start with general appearance and vital signs.

- Measure length, weight, and FOC (frontal-occipital circumference). Calculate whether the neonate is AGA, SGA, or LGA by converting the raw data into percentiles.

- Approximate the gestational age of the neonate. Use the estimated date of confinement (EDC) that the obstetricians defined, whether based on last menstrual period (LMP), early ultrasound, or both, along with the gestational age of the neonate you have calculated using the Ballard Score. This method utilizes a set of pre-defined criteria with the physical examination designed to deliver a score that estimates the approximate gestational age at delivery.

You should perform a complete physical examination on every newborn you admit (see Appendix F: The Normal Newborn Examination), and, during the oral case presentation report pertinent normal and abnormal findings.

Step 6: Provide the results of laboratory studies / other studies. Usual studies drawn at birth include blood type and Rh status.

- Other studies drawn at birth for high-risk infants include a CBC with differential, Coombs test, etc.

- Electrolytes, when needed, are typically first sent at 12-24 hours of life, unless the neonate is receiving critical care.

- Glucose levels are tested as clinically indicated for infants at risk for hypoglycemia.

Be sure to have the most up-to-date version of the laboratory data.

Diagnostic imaging studies—such as radiography, ECG, or echocardiogram studies—are performed as clinically indicated.

Should your patient have any abnormal laboratory or other test results, discuss the significance of these results with the intern or resident prior to your presentation. This will allow critical laboratory or other test results to be considered and their underlying causes to be treated earlier and allow you a chance to try out your interpretation of the result—and the ensuing plan— before your presentation to the attending pediatrician.

Step 7: Give the assessment and plan.

● Begin with a statement of one or two sentences summarizing the patient and the patient's problems.

● For every item on the patient's problem list, a differential diagnosis ranked in order of likelihood should be given.

● Give an organized clinical plan of care for each of the patient's problems.

Mistake #96

Not discussing pertinent obstetrical and perinatal events

As discussed above, the medical history of a neonate largely consists of the mother's pregnancy history and the events surrounding the baby's delivery. Therefore, it is imperative that you know and relay this information to the rest of the nursery team for proper patient care.

Chapter 17

Commonly Made Mistakes On

The Daily Progress Note (Nursery)

In general, daily nursery progress notes are similar to daily progress notes written on older pediatric patients in the hospital (see Chapter 6). Commonly made mistakes on the daily progress note that are particular to the nursery, however, are discussed below.

Mistake **#97**

Not documenting the patient's exact age on every progress note

It is important to know the exact day of life for the patient. The differential diagnosis and management of certain diseases such as sepsis or conditions such as jaundice are influenced by the patient's precise age, sometimes even by the hour.

Success tip #72

In addition to documenting the patient's exact age on your progress note, include the post-gestational age. For example,

"DOL #2 (post-gestational age 38 4/7 weeks)."

Mistake #98

Not documenting the patient's exact weight on every progress note

Knowing the patient's exact weight in kilograms is vital to proper patient care in neonatology. As medication dosages, caloric goals, feeding schedules, and ins and outs for the neonate are all calculated based on weight in kilograms, it is imperative to obtain and document the exact daily weight on every progress note.

Success tip #73

In addition to documenting the daily weight in your progress note, indicate how much weight was gained or lost from both the previous day and the baby's birth weight, in grams and percentage. For example, one might write the following:

"Weight today is 4100 grams—an 85 gram, or ~2%, decrease from yesterday and a 185 gram, or ~4.4%, decrease from the birth weight of 4285 grams."

Mistake #99

Not documenting specific age-related changes in the physical examination

Many aspects of the neonatal physical examination will change during the first week of life. The cardiovascular system in particular is in a dynamic state during the first week of like, which is often reflected by the presence or absence of murmurs heard on auscultation during the physical examination. For example, the ductus arteriosus murmur often is heard on the first day of life, but may disappear by the second day of life as the ductus closes functionally. Carefully perform a complete physical examination of the neonate every day, and clearly document your findings in the daily progress note.

Mistake #100

Not documenting the date(s) of completion or failure of routine newborn screening

Routine neonatal screening includes the newborn screen and a hearing screen prior to patient discharge. Although the exact content of the newborn screen varies from state to state, all 50 states, the District of Columbia, Puerto Rico, and the US Virgin Islands provide universal screening of newborns for PKU and congenital hypothyroidism. Most states additionally screen for galactosemia and hemoglobinopathies; in addition, some states include testing for maple syrup urine disease, homocystinuria, biotinidase deficiency, congenital adrenal hyperplasia, cystic fibrosis, and tyrosinemia. For normal newborns, the state newborn screen is obtained as close to hospital discharge as possible; if the state newborn screen is obtained at less than 24 hours of life, a repeat state newborn screen is performed at one to two weeks of life. In addition to the state newborn screen, a hearing screen performed by either an OAE (otoacoustic emission) test or an ABR (auditory brainstem response) test is also usually performed on newborns prior to hospital discharge. Although the results of the state newborn screen may not be available by the time the newborn leaves the hospital, the results of the hearing screen will be—and need to be documented. The American Academy of Pediatrics Task Force on Newborn

and Infant Screening currently recommends that all
newborns have hearing screening before the age of one
month, with audiologic confirmation of hearing loss by
three months for those newborns that failed their initial
screen, and intervention by six months.

Success tip #74

Determine which diseases are screened for in your
state's newborn screen by visiting
http://genes-r-us.uthscsa.edu.

Success tip #75

Familiarize yourself with the differences between the
OAE and ABR hearing screening tests and their
indications.

Success tip #76

Discuss with your team the indications for other types
of pre-hospital discharge tests for newborns such as
car seat testing and vision testing.

Chapter 18

Commonly Made Mistakes During

Attending Rounds (Nursery)

In general, attending rounds in the nursery are similar to pediatric attending rounds in other locations of the hospital (see Chapter 7). Commonly made mistakes during attending rounds that are particular to the nursery, however, are discussed below.

Mistake **#101**

Not understanding the clinical significance of illness on a neonate's growth and development

Pediatrics is a medical specialty focused on growth and development starting with day-of-life one. Illnesses acquired and combated during a neonate's first few days of life can have a significant impact on their subsequent maturation. Discuss with the medical team and the attending pediatrician the potential impact of a newborn's illness on their future growth and development. Understanding the potential significance of an illness on the newborn will not only increase your knowledge as a physician-in-training, but will also—and more importantly—alert you to the stress and tension a family endures when dealing with a sick newborn. In these instances, the power of empathy should never be underestimated.

APPENDIX A: 10 TIPS FOR SUCCESS

1 Prior to starting the rotation, ask other medical students who have completed the rotation for advice.

2 Make sure you have all the appropriate equipment prior to the start of the rotation. For pediatrics, you should carry the following equipment with you:

- Stethoscope, with pediatric bell and diaphragm, if available
- Ophthalmoscope, for evaluating the red reflex
- Otoscope with pneumatic attachment, for viewing and evaluating the mobility of the tympanic membrane
- Calculator, as most pediatric medications are dosed in mg/kg
- Reflex hammer
- Measuring tape, for measuring head circumference, etc.
- Tongue blades
- Penlight
- Pens
- Toy, for distracting apprehensive children
- Books, electronic and/or printed

3 Have a pocket reference book available with normal pediatric laboratory values based on age.

4 Take notes on teaching points made by your fellow students, interns, residents, and attendings. Review your notes at the end of each day rather than just filing them.

5 Read about your patient's problems and diagnoses. By doing this, you will not only understand more about the pathophysiology of the disease process and its treatment, but you will be prepared to ask more intelligible questions regarding patient management.

6 Bring your team a nice handout whenever you give a talk/presentation.

7 On rounds, state ins as follows: (1) type of 'in' (breastfeeding, breastmilk by bottle, formula by bottle, orogastric feeds); and (2) amount of 'in' in terms of mL/kg/day (e.g., Enfamil® PO by bottle at 100 mL/kg/day; or breastfeeding PO ad lib plus Enfamil® PO by bottle at 60 mL/kg/day, with D5W + NaCl 2 mEq/100mL + KCl 2 mEq/100mL at 40 mL/kg/day).

8 State urine output (UOP) as mL/kg/hr.

9 Know your patient's immunization status.

10 Remember that breast milk is 20 kcal/oz.

APPENDIX B: INTERPRETING THE PEDIATRIC ECG

Although electrocardiograms (ECGs) are ordered far less frequently in pediatric medicine than in adult medicine, it is nevertheless important to have a basic understanding of their reading and interpretation. The ECG computer is usually reliable when it comes to calculating heart rate and ECG intervals—with the exception of the corrected QT interval (see below). However, the interpretation of the ECG that is often printed on the top of the electrocardiogram should not always be taken at face value as the ECG machines are usually programmed to interpret adult tracings, and therefore are frequently incorrect in the tracing interpretation of a pediatric patient.

An example of a systematic approach to interpreting a pediatric ECG is discussed below.

Step-by-step approach to the interpretation of the pediatric ECG

Step 1: Note identifying information, including the patient name and medical record number on the ECG. Determine the exact age of the patient. This will be *essential* when interpreting ECG data against age-specific reference ranges. Follow this by noting the time and date of the tracing.

Step 2: Determine the rationale/reason for obtaining the ECG. Was this a patient with chest pain or a newborn with a newly diagnosed heart murmur? Is this a patient with known congenital heart disease? Did the patient have a syncopal event or an apneic episode?

Step 3: Determine the heart rate. There are multiple approaches to this task. Two are as follows:

Method 1

With a routine recording speed of 25 mm/sec, each mm = 0.04 sec, and each 5 mm division (the distance between two heavy lines) = 0.20 sec. Thus, every 5 large divisions = 1 sec.

Look for the dark "tick" marks above the tracing. These occur every 15 large divisions, or 3 sec.

For fast heart rates, count the number of R waves within 15 large divisions (3 sec), and multiply that number by 20, to arrive at the number of beats in one minute. For slower heart rates, perform your count over 30 large divisions, or 6 sec, and multiply that number by 10.

Method 2

The heart rate can also be approximated by memorizing selected heart rates for given RR intervals. The RR interval is the distance between successive R waves on the ECG.

For best approximation, choose an R wave that appears on, or near, a large division (heavier line) on the ECG.

When RR intervals are 5, 10, 15, 20, and 25 mm, the heart rates are 300, 150, 100, 75, 60, and 50 beats per minute (bpm), respectively. (In other words, the heart rate parallels 300 divided by the number of heavy lines).

Compare the determined heart rate with age-specific norms (see following table).

Age	HR range (mean)
0 – 1 mo	100-160 (130)
1 mo – 6 mo	100-180 (145)
6 mo – 1 yr	100-170 (135)
1 yr – 3 yr	90-150 (120)

4 yr – 8 yr	65-135 (110)
9 yr – 16 yr	60-110 (85)
> 16 yr	60-100 (80)

Step 4: Identify the rhythm. More often than not, the basic rhythm in pediatric patients will be normal sinus rhythm; however, this is not always the case. To classify the rhythm as normal sinus, there must be (1) an identifiable P wave prior to every QRS complex, (2) a QRS complex after every P wave, and (3) a normal P wave axis (between 0 and +90 degrees—in other words, upright P waves in leads I and aVF). Refer to a pediatric ECG-specific text for a more advanced discussion of pediatric rhythm analysis.

Step 5: Identify the QRS axis. The P wave axis should already have been determined, above. By looking at leads I and aVF, the QRS axis may then be determined, or, more routinely, located within one of the four basic quadrants on the ECG (0 to +90, +90 to ±180, 0 to -90, or -90 to ±180 degrees) (see table below).

Lead I (mean QRS deflection)	Lead aVF (mean QRS deflection)	Mean Axis (degrees)
Positive (+)	Positive (+)	0 to +90 (normal axis)
Positive (+)	Negative (-)	0 to -90 (leftward axis)
Negative (-)	Positive (+)	+90 to ±180 (rightward axis)
Negative (-)	Negative (-)	-90 to ±180 (indeterminate axis)

In newborns it can be entirely normal to have a rightward axis, whereas in adults one would be concerned for right ventricular hypertrophy or pulmonary hypertension, as the pulmonary pressures in neonates remain elevated for the first few weeks of life.

Compare the determined QRS axis with age-specific norms (see table below).

Age	QRS axis (mean)
0 – 1 mo	+30 to ±180 (+110)
1 mo – 6 mo	+10 to +125 (+70)
6 mo – 1 yr	+10 to +125 (+60)
1 yr – 3 yr	+10 to +125 (+60)
4 yr – 8 yr	0 to +110 (+60)
9 yr – 16 yr	-15 to +110 (+60)
> 16 yr	-15 to +110 (+60)

It is not considered "normal" in a neonate to have a superior axis—that is, an axis between 0 and ±180 degrees. Etiologies of a superior axis in a newborn include endocardial cushion defects (such as a common AV canal), tricuspid atresia, and Noonan syndrome.

Step 6: Calculate the intervals, durations, and segments (all of which are age- and heart rate-dependent). The table below shows normal age-specific parameters for the PR interval and QRS duration.

Age	PR interval (sec)	QRS duration (sec)
0 – 1 mo	0.08-0.12 (0.10)	0.05 (0.07)
1 mo – 6 mo	0.08-0.13 (0.11)	0.05 (0.07)
6 mo – 1 yr	0.10-0.14 (0.12)	0.05 (0.07)

1 yr – 3 yr	0.10-0.14 (0.12)	0.06 (0.07)
4 yr – 8 yr	0.11-0.15 (0.13)	0.07 (0.08)
9 yr – 16 yr	0.12-0.17 (0.14)	0.07 (0.09)
> 16 yr	0.12-0.20 (0.15)	0.08 (0.10)
Mean values for PR interval and QRS duration are in parentheses.		

Heart Block

If the PR interval is prolonged, consider heart block, which can be one of the following:

1st degree
2nd degree type 1 (Wenckebach)
2nd degree type 2 (Mobitz, High Grade AV block)
3rd degree (Complete AV block)

Wolff-Parkinson-White Syndrome

If the PR interval is < 0.08 mm, consider the Wolff-Parkinson-White (WPW) syndrome. In this syndrome, there is typically both a short PR interval in addition to an up-sloping of the PR segment (the so-called delta wave, which fades into the normally almost-vertical waves of the QRS complex), both of which suggest the presence of an electrical bypass tract. In the presence of a bypass tract, electrical signals originating in the atria are not subject to the proper "conduction delay" at the AV node and pass rapidly via an atypical conduction pathway to the ventricles.

The QTc, or the QT segment corrected for the heart rate, is calculated as the QT segment divided by the square root of the preceding RR interval:

$$QTc = QT \text{ (sec)} / \sqrt{R\text{-}R \text{ (sec)}}$$

Always calculate the QTc yourself (do *not* use the computer-derived value), and then compare your calculated QTc with age-specific norms.

Age	Normal QTc (sec)
Infants	0.45
Children	0.44
Adults	0.42

A prolonged QTc can be seen in the presence of hypocalcemia, hypokalemia, hypomagnesemia, myocarditis, the long QT syndrome, head injury, or toxicity from quinidine, procainamide, phenothiazines, and tricyclic antidepressants.

A shortened QTc can be seen with hypercalcemia, digoxin, phenytoin, and propranolol.

Step 7: Assess for the presence of atrial and ventricular hypertrophy. In lead II, the presence of an abnormally tall P wave (> 2.5 mm) suggests right atrial hypertrophy (or enlargement), whereas the presence of an abnormally wide P wave (> 2.5 mm) suggests left atrial hypertrophy (or enlargement). A biphasic P wave in lead V1 is also suggestive of left atrial enlargement. In terms of ventricular enlargement, right ventricular hypertrophy (RVH) is suggested by the findings of right axis deviation (RAD), a large (increased amplitude) R wave in V1, and a deep (large negative amplitude) S wave in V6. A positive (upright) T wave in lead V1 between the ages of 1 week and adolescence is also suggestive of RVH. Left ventricular hypertrophy (LVH) is suggested by the presence of a deep S wave in V1 and a large R wave in V6. ECG evidence of volume overload (e.g., Q waves > 5 mm and tall T waves in V5 or V6) is also suggestive of LVH.

See the following tables for normative age-specific R and S wave amplitudes for leads V1 and V6.

Lead V1:

Age	R wave amplitude (mm)	S wave amplitude (mm)	R/S ratio
0 – 1 mo	12 (24)	6.5 (20)	2.5
1 mo – 6 mo	10 (19)	5.5 (15)	2.3
6 mo – 1 yr	9.5 (20)	6.5 (18)	1.6
1 yr – 3 yr	8.5 (18)	9 (20)	1.2
4 yr – 8 yr	7 (15)	11 (22)	0.7
9 yr – 16 yr	5 (12)	11 (22)	0.5
> 16 yr	3 (9)	10 (20)	0.3

Numbers are expressed as mean values and, in parentheses, 98th percentile

Lead V6:

Age	R wave amplitude (mm)	S wave amplitude (mm)	R/S ratio
0 – 1 mo	5.5 (14)	3.5 (9.5)	3.0
1 mo – 6 mo	12.5 (22)	2.5 (8.5)	5.5
6 mo – 1 yr	12.5 (22.5)	2 (7.5)	7.5
1 yr – 3 yr	14 (23.5)	1.5 (6)	10
4 yr – 8 yr	16 (26)	1 (4.5)	13
9 yr - 16 yr	15 (25)	1 (4)	14.5
> 16 yr	10 (20)	0.8 (4)	12

Numbers are expressed as mean values and, in parentheses, 98th percentile

Step 8: Assess the repolarization pattern represented by the T waves on the ECG. A normal ECG in the early post-natal period demonstrates upright T waves in lead V1. This T wave (in V1) subsequently "flips" some time around the first week of life, and remains negative until some time in adolescence, when the T wave in V1 again becomes positive, or upright. Thus, an upright T wave in lead V1 in a four-year-old is considered *abnormal* (and suggestive of RVH, as discussed above). Compare the T wave axis with age-specific norms (see tables below).

Age	T wave – Leads V1 and V2	T wave – Lead aVF	T wave – Leads I, V5, and V6
Birth – 1 day	±	+	±
1 day – 4 days	±	+	+
4 days – adolescence	-	+	+
Adolescence – adulthood	+	+	+

ST-segment elevation or depression is suggestive of myocardial injury.

Tall T waves are suggestive of hyperkalemia or left ventricular hypertrophy.

Flattened T waves are suggestive of hypothyroidism, hypokalemia, pericarditis, myocarditis, and myocardial ischemia. T waves can also be relatively flat in the presence of digoxin, and in the normal newborn ECG.

U waves (usually associated with hypokalemia) are not necessarily abnormal findings; in fact, an accentuated U wave is normal in the newborn ECG.

Step 9: Compare the current ECG to a previous ECG (or ECGs) from the same patient, if available. This is key to describing interval changes. The comparison will also help you assess what is "normal" for this patient and what (if anything) has changed from a previous baseline examination.

Step-by-step approach to the pediatric ECG interpretation

Step 1: Note identifying information.

Step 2: Determine the rationale/reason for obtaining the ECG.

Step 3: Determine the heart rate.

Step 4: Identify the rhythm.

Step 5: Identify the QRS axis.

Step 6: Calculate the intervals, durations, and segments.

Step 7: Assess for the presence of atrial and ventricular hypertrophy.

Step 8: Assess the repolarization pattern.

Step 9: Compare the current ECG to a previous ECG.

APPENDIX C: INTERPRETING THE PEDIATRIC CHEST RADIOGRAPH

Many will tell you that it is good practice to review the reading of a radiological study with a radiologist—and it is. Nevertheless, you should read each chest radiograph (CXR) initially on your own. Practice reading each radiograph in a systematic and orderly manner. An example of a helpful method is given below.

No matter how obvious a parenchymal lesion may be, always examine the film as well for any lines or tubes (nasogastric tubes, central lines, endotracheal tubes), the integrity of the bones, the characteristics of the diaphragm, the position of the trachea, and the other anatomical structures in the chest.

Every attending radiologist has a story to tell about an on-call radiologist who read the CXR as "left lower lobe infiltrate consistent with pneumonia" but failed to take note of the broken clavicle and humerus, which might have suggested the diagnosis of abuse—only to see the child return subsequently with a fractured skull, or worse. The order of your systematic approach to evaluating the CXR is not important, but having a systematic approach is vital.

Step-by-step approach to the interpretation of the pediatric CXR

Step 1: Note identifying information, including the patient's name and medical record number on the CXR (regardless of whether the film is a digital or print version). Determine the time and date of the study to ensure that you are interpreting the correct film.

Step 2: Determine the rationale/reason for ordering the CXR. Was this chest film ordered as a routine pre-operative screen or for a child with shortness of breath?

Is there an underlying chronic disease that might affect
the pulmonary parenchyma or interstitium such as
asthma or cystic fibrosis? Or, alternatively, was the study
ordered merely to verify the correct location of a medical
device or catheter after placement? Regardless of the
reason, one needs to know the indication for the proper
interpretation of the chest radiograph.

**Step 3: Describe the type of film, position of the
patient, and quality of the radiograph.** A full CXR
series will be obtained as PA (postero-anterior, or from
back to front) and lateral films. The "PA film" name
suggests the direction the x-ray beam travels—from the
patient's back → to his or her front → to the film
cassette anterior to the chest wall. This is in contrast to
the "AP film," which is generally obtained with a portable
radiograph device. Other chest radiograph positions
include supine or semi-supine (flat on the back or at an
upright angle but not fully erect), as well as left or right
lateral decubitus (lying on the left or right side).

Although not intentional positions, patients may also be
described as rotated (typically to the right or left side) on
the film, a finding which may alter your interpretation of
various findings to some extent. Utilize the appearance of
the clavicles in order to assess for patient rotation.
Radiographs are obtained under a wide variety of
conditions, technical properties and limitations, all of
which are far beyond the technical capacity of this text,
but the result of which are films of varying quality and
exposure.

Films that appear "too white" are more appropriately
described as "under penetrated." Think of the whole film
looking like bone, which appears white because it is very
dense, thus not allowing many x-rays to pass through it
to reach the cassette. In an under penetrated film, the
vertebrae cannot be identified behind the heart.

In contrast to under-penetrated films are films that appear "too black" or, more appropriately, are "over penetrated." Think of the lungs, which are full of low density air, and thus allow many x-rays to pass through to reach the film cassette. In over-penetrated films, pulmonary vessels cannot be fully differentiated in the lung periphery.

Step 4: Assess the adequacy of inspiration. To best determine the degree of patient inspiration, count the number of posterior ribs; a good inspiratory film will reveal ten posterior ribs. If the CXR is taken with a poor inspiratory effort by the patient, the lungs will look like they have small volumes, and the heart may looked "squished" and possibly large in comparison to the rest of the chest. It may also appear as if the patient has an interstitial process occurring secondary to poor chest expansion. Poor inspiratory films are difficult to interpret, and should as a rule be re-taken with the patient giving a better inspiratory effort.

Having said that, neonates and infants will not be able to follow instructions and cooperate with deep inspiration on command, so do what you can and interpret the CXR of a neonate or infant taking into account the possible limitations of the film secondary to poor inspiratory effort.

Step 5: Detail all lines, tubes, ports, drains, sponges, hardware, or other medical devices seen on the CXR. Be as specific as possible in describing the device and noting its apparent location. The lateral projection will aid you in your three dimensional localization of the device or foreign object.

Step 6: Describe the visible bony anatomy, looking for evidence of fracture, bone disease or lesion, and overall homogeneity of the bone evident on the chest radiograph. In pediatrics, fractures at the physis (growth plate) may present in the form of one of five distinct lesions, known collectively as the Salter-Harris or Salter classification. In simple terms, the Salter classification can be broken down as follows:

I   **S**ALTER I: **S**lipped physis. Look for evidence of a widening of the physis (separation of the epiphysis from the metaphysis).

II   S**A**LTER II: Fracture involves the physis as well as the bone **A**bove or proximal to the epiphysis. The Salter-Harris type II fractures are the most common types of growth plate fractures.

III   SA**L**TER III: Fracture involves the physis as well as the bone be**L**ow or distal to the epiphysis. In this type of fracture, the fracture crosses the growth plate, and bone growth may be arrested.

IV   SAL**T**ER IV: Fracture extends **T**hrough the physis, involving bone both proximal and distal to the epiphyseal plate. The fracture line runs through the epiphysis, physis, and the metaphysis.

V   SALTE**R** V: A w**R**ecked—crushed or compressed—growth plate, where the physeal space has been severely reduced or narrowed. It may appear as if there is no physis on the side of the injury. Careful examination, however, will show evidence of an open growth plate on the contralateral side.

Evidence of fracture may also present well after the initial trauma in the form of a healing callus at the site of injury. Detailing the bony anatomy should also include a survey of the anterior and posterior ribs, as fractures here may provide evidence of ongoing or past child abuse. It is unlikely that a child who is too young to walk could develop a long bone fracture on his or her own.

Step 7: Describe the soft tissue, looking for evidence of edema, lesions, or asymmetry. The soft tissue should not appear overly calcified. In the appropriate clinical setting or after a trauma, evaluate the film for subcutaneous emphysema.

Step 8: Analyze the cardiac borders for evidence of infiltrate or lesion. The right and left heart borders should appear sharp; a loss of this normal sharpness suggests a nearby lesion in the adjacent lung parenchyma. Knowing one's pulmonary anatomy is key: lesions overlying the right heart border are classically in the right middle lobe (RML), while lesions overlying the left heart border are typically lingular, the equivalent of a left middle lobe, in origin.

The cardiac shadow may also be examined for evidence of cardiomegaly, typically described as a cardiac shadow extending for greater than 50% of the width and depth of the thorax on the PA and lateral projections, respectively. AP films should not be utilized to assess for the presence of cardiac enlargement as they tend to increase the apparent size of the heart secondary to technical reasons. Think of where the x-ray originates and which objects might be magnified. Meanwhile, don't be tricked by the nuances of a pediatric chest film. The appearance of the still-present thymus gland is similar in density to the heart, often fooling new students into over-calling cardiomegaly. Consider describing the heart borders as the "cardio-thymic silhouette."

Step 9: Continue analyzing borders by visualizing the cardiophrenic and costophrenic angles as well as the hemi-diaphragms for evidence of infiltrate or effusion. Loss of a clean right cardiophrenic angle or right hemi-

diaphragm (see the lateral projection for confirmation)
suggest right lower lobe (RLL) lesions, while similar
radiographic changes on the contralateral side suggest
lesions in or around the left lower lobe (LLL). In over 90%
of patients, the normal right hemi-diaphragm is elevated
above the position of the left hemi-diaphragm, due at
least in part to the presence of the liver. Blunting of either
costophrenic angle implicates a possible pleural process,
most typically suggesting a pleural effusion. If this is the
case, look for a meniscus.

**Step 10: Describe the appearance of the
mediastinum and any visible structures.** Note the
position of the trachea, midline or otherwise. Describe
any lesions, should they be present. If not done above,
evaluate the appropriateness of the thymus and
pulmonary vasculature. Be sure to also examine the
hilum, particularly looking for hilar lymphadenopathy (TB,
sarcoidosis, etc.).

**Step 11: Examine the lung parenchyma and
interstitial spaces** for evidence of pulmonary pathology.
As a general rule, visible fissures suggest the presence
of fluid. Follow the lung markings out to the periphery,
especially in the apices of the lungs; absence of lung
markings suggests the presence of a pneumothorax.
Look for evidence of consolidative (usually unilateral and
single-lobed) versus interstitial (usually bilateral involving
several lobes) processes. Always compare the right lung
fields to the left lung fields; in a patient without pulmonary
disease, the general appearance of the lung fields should
be similar. In the right clinical setting, examine the film for
cephalization (if you are concerned about heart failure),
nodules (if you are concerned about chemical
exposures), or granulomas (if you are concerned about
infectious and/or infiltrative processes). Also note the
caliber of the pleura, as many disease processes can
cause pleural thickening.

Step 12: Compare the current film to a previous film (or films) from the same patient, if available. This is key to describing interval changes. The comparison will also help you assess what is "normal" for this patient and what (if anything) has changed from a previous baseline examination.

Step-by-step approach to the pediatric CXR interpretation

Step 1: Note identifying information.

Step 2: Determine the rationale/reason for ordering the CXR.

Step 3: Describe the type of film, position of the patient, and quality of the radiograph.

Step 4: Assess the adequacy of inspiration.

Step 5: Detail all lines, tubes, ports, drains, sponges, hardware, or other medical devices.

Step 6: Describe the visible bony anatomy.

Step 7: Describe the soft tissue.

Step 8: Analyze the cardiac borders.

Step 9: Continue analyzing borders by visualizing the cardiophrenic and costophrenic angles as well as the hemi-diaphragms.

Step 10: Describe the appearance of the mediastinum and any visible structures.

Step 11: Examine the lung parenchyma and interstitial spaces.

Step 12: Compare the current film to a previous film.

Appendix D: Types of Commonly Used Infant and Pediatric Formulas

Formulas are usually classified based on (1) age of the recipient (premature neonate, neonate, infant, child, or adult), and (2) composition (protein, carbohydrate, fat). We have included information below on the composition of pediatric formulas, both standard and specialized, for infants (birth - 1 year), young children (1 - 10 years), and older children (> 10 years).

Unless otherwise specified, infant formulas are 20 kcal/oz (similar to breastmilk). However, some premature neonate formulas are concentrated to 24 kcal/oz. Many supplements such as Enfacare® are also available to increase the caloric content of standard formulas. Formulas that include the words "Lipil" or "Advance" usually contain a specialized blend of docosahexaenoic acid (DHA) and arachidonic acid (ARA). In addition, most formulas are fortified with iron.

Standard Infant Formulas (birth - 1 year)

Formula	Protein	Carbohydrate	Fat	Indication for use
Similac®, Enfamil®	Whole cow milk,* (casein, whey)	Lactose	Soy, coconut, safflower, ± sunflower, palm	Normal GI tract
Similac Lactose Free®, Enfamil Lactofree®	Whole cow milk,* (casein, whey)	Corn syrup solids ± sucrose	Soy, coconut, safflower, ± sunflower, palm	Lactose malabsorption
Isomil®, ProSobee®	Soy#	Corn syrup solids ± sucrose	Soy, coconut, ± sunflower, safflower, palm	Allergy to cow's milk, lactose malabsorption, galactosemia

*Whole cow milk protein formulas (with iron) are the standard of care for infant formula feeding.

#Soy formulas are an alternative for infant formula feeding for documented cow milk protein sensitivity or lactose intolerance. *(Approximately 50% of infants with documented cow milk protein sensitivity will be sensitive to soy protein as well, and will thus require a specialized infant formula).*

Specialized Infant Formulas (birth - 1 year)

Formula	Protein	Carbohydrate	Fat	Indication for use
Alimentum®	Casein hydrolysate*	Tapioca starch, sucrose	Soy, safflower, medium chain triglyceride (MCT)	Food allergies, protein or fat malabsorption
Pregestimil®	Casein hydrolysate*	Corn syrup solids, cornstarch, dextrose	Soy, safflower, corn, MCT	Food allergies, protein or fat malabsorption

Nutramigen®	Casein hydrolysate*	Corn syrup solids, cornstarch	Soy, coconut, sunflower, palm (NO MCT)	Food allergies
Good Start®	Whey hydrolysate*	Lactose, maltodextrin	Safflower, coconut, soy, palm	Normal GI tract
Neocate®	Amino acids#	Corn syrup solids	Safflower, coconut, soy	Severe food allergies

*Protein hydrolysate formulas are a therapeutic formula for infants with documented cow milk and soy protein sensitivity or malabsorption syndromes.
#Amino acid formulas are a therapeutic formula for infants with documented protein hydrolysate sensitivity or allergic gastroenteropathy.

Standard Pediatric Formulas (1-10 years)*				
Formula	Protein	Carbohydrate	Fat	Indication for use
PediaSure® (1 kcal/mL)	Caseinates, whey	Maltodextrin, sucrose	Safflower, soy, MCT	Normal GI tract (oral or tube feed)
Kindercal® (1 kcal/mL)	Milk protein concentrate	Maltodextrin, sucrose	Sunflower, canola, corn, MCT	Normal GI tract (oral or tube feed)
Nutren Jr® (1 kcal/mL)	Caseinates, whey	Maltodextrin, sucrose	Soy, canola, MCT	Normal GI tract (oral or tube feed)

*Standard pediatric formulas are used for dietary supplementation in children with poor weight gain or for the sole source of enteral nutrition in children with feeding disorders or chronic diseases.

Specialized Pediatric Formulas (1 - 10 years)*

Formula	Protein	Carbohy-drate	Fat	Indication for use
Peptamen Jr® (1 kcal/mL)	Hydrolyzed whey	Maltodextrin, corn starch, sucrose	Canola, soy, MCT	Malabsorption syndromes (oral or tube feed)
NeocateOne+® (1 kcal/mL)	Amino acids	Corn syrup solids	Safflower, canola, MCT	Malabsorption syndromes or protein allergies (oral or tube feed)

*Specialized pediatric formulas are used for the sole source of enteral nutrition in children with documented cow milk or soy protein sensitivity or malabsorption syndromes.

Standard Older Child Formulas (> 10 years)*

Formula	Protein	Carbohy-drate	Fat	Indication for use
Boost® (1 kcal/mL)	Milk protein concentrate	Corn syrup solids, sucrose	Sunflower, corn, canola	Oral supplement
Ensure® (1 kcal/mL)	Caseinates, whey	Maltodextrin, corn syrup solids, sucrose	Safflower, corn, canola	Oral supplement or tube feeding with normal GI tract

*Standard older child formulas are used for dietary supplementation in children with poor weight gain or for the sole source of enteral nutrition in children with feeding disorders or chronic diseases.

Specialized Older Child Formulas (> 10 years)*

Formula	Protein	Carbohydrate	Fat	Indication for use
Peptamen® (1 kcal/mL)	Hydrolyzed whey	Maltodextrin, corn starch	Soybean, MCT	Malabsorption syndromes
Nepro® (2 kcal/mL)	Caseinates	Corn syrup solids, sucrose, fructose, oligosaccharides	Safflower, canola, lecithin	Renal failure
Glucerna® (1 kcal/mL)	Caseinates	Maltodextrin, soy, fructose	Safflower, canola, lecithin	Impaired glucose tolerance

*Specialized older child formulas are used for the sole source of enteral nutrition in children with documented cow milk or soy protein sensitivity, malabsorption syndromes, or specific chronic diseases.

Formulas Used Predominantly for Tube Feeding (1- 10 years)

Formula	Protein	Carbohydrate	Fat	Indication for use
PediaSure® (1 kcal/mL)	Caseinates, whey	Maltodextrin, sucrose	Safflower, soy, MCT	Normal GI tract
Nutren Jr® (1 kcal/mL)	Caseinates, whey	Maltodextrin, sucrose	Soy, canola, MCT	Normal GI tract
Kindercal TF® (1 kcal/mL)	Milk protein concentrate	Maltodextrin, sucrose	Sunflower, canola, corn, MCT	Normal GI tract

Formulas Used Predominantly for Tube Feeding (> 10 years)

Formula	Protein	Carbohy-drate	Fat	Indication for use
Ensure® (1 kcal/mL)	Caseinates, whey	Maltodextrin, corn syrup solids, sucrose	Safflower, corn, canola	Normal GI tract
Osmolite® (1 kcal/mL)	Caseinates, soy	Maltodextrin	Safflower, canola, lecithin, MCT	Normal GI tract
Isocal® (1 kcal/mL)	Caseinates, soy	Maltodextrin	Soy, MCT	Normal GI tract
Nutren 2.0® (2 kcal/mL)	Caseinates	Corn syrup solids, maltodextrin, sucrose	Canola, corn, lecithin, MCT	Increased caloric needs, fluid restriction

APPENDIX E: TYPES OF ORAL REHYDRATION SOLUTIONS

Product	Carbohydrate (g/L)	Osmolality (mOsm)
Enfalyte®	Rice syrup solids (30)	200
Oral Rehydration Salts (ORS)®	Dextrose (20)	330
Pedialyte®	Dextrose (25)	250
Rehydralyte®	Dextrose (25)	305

APPENDIX F: THE NORMAL NEWBORN EXAMINATION

The newborn examination should be performed in the following order:

1. Observation
2. Auscultation of the chest (with a warm stethoscope)
3. Palpation of the abdomen
4. Examination of the head, ears, eyes, nose, throat, genitalia, hips, extremities, and reflexes (performed last as these are most likely to irritate the neonate)

Listed in the table below are certain aspects of the physical examination pertinent to the neonate.

Physical examination of the normal newborn	
Component of physical examination	Check for...
Skin	Bruising, petechiae, birthmarks, hemangiomas, nevi, café au lait spots, rashes, edema, pallor, cyanosis, and jaundice. Also note the presence or absence of meconium staining and/or lanugo.
Head	Cephalohematoma, caput succedaneum, or subgaleal hemorrhages. Also evaluate the size and presence of fontanelles and suture alignment. In addition, look carefully at the neonate to check for odd facies such as syndromic facies.

Face	Odd facies (syndromic facies).
Ears	Malformed or malpositioned ears. Also check for pre-auriciular malformations such as pits and/or tags.
Eyes	Subconjunctival hemorrhages and iris abnormalities. Always check for a bilateral red reflex.
Nose	Choanal atresia. (Remember, neonates under 1 month of age are obligate nose breathers.)
Mouth	Retention cysts (Epstein pearls) and neonatal teeth. Also check the tongue and the integrity and shape of the palate.
Neck	Redundant skin or webbing, sinus tracts, and masses.
Chest & Lungs	Fractured clavicles and equal and symmetric breath sounds.
Heart	Normal heart sounds and murmurs.
Abdomen	Softness, distension, bowel sounds, and for possible masses and/or deformities.
Genitalia & Anus	Descended testicles (males); in females, check the condition of the vulva. In both sexes, check for hernias and for a patent anus.
Skeleton	Obvious abnormalities and hip integrity. Also evaluate carefully for arthrogryposis, neural tube defects, and spinal dysraphisms.
Neurologic examination	Neonatal reflexes, including sucking reflex, rooting reflex, traction response, palmar grasp, placing reflex, moro (startle) reflex, and tonic neck reflex.

APPENDIX G: AGE-APPROPRIATE DEVELOPMENTAL MILESTONES

Age	Gross motor	Visual-motor/ problem solving	Language	Personal/ social
1 mo	Raises head from prone position	Tracks horizontally to midline	Alerts to sound	Regards face
2 mo	Raises chest from prone position	Tracks horizontally past midline; tracks vertically	Social smile	Recognizes parent
3 mo	Supports weight on forearms; holds head up steadily	Tracks 360°; hands unfisted	Coos	Reaches for familiar objects/ people
4 mo	Rolls prone to supine; supports weight in prone position on wrists (with arms straight)	Brings hands to midline; reaches with arms in unison towards objects	Orients to voice; laughs aloud	Looks around inquisitively
5 mo	Rolls supine to prone	Reaches up for objects while supine	Orients to sound	Works for a toy

6 mo	Sits unsupported; puts feet in mouth when supine	Transfers objects from hand-to-hand, raking grasp, unilateral reach	Babbles; ah-goo; razzes	Stranger recognition
9 mo	Crawls; cruises; pulls to stand	Immature pincer grasp; rings bell; probes with forefinger; throws objects	Says "mama" and "dada" non-specifically; understands "no"; waves bye-bye	Plays gesture games (e.g., pat-a-cake); explorative
12 mo	Walks alone with independent steps	Mature pincer grasp; intentional release; uses crayon	Uses 2 words other than "mama/dada"; follows 1-step gestured command	Comes when called; imitates actions of others
15 mo	Walks backwards; creeps up stairs	Scribbles in imitation; builds tower of 2 blocks	Uses 4-6 words; follows 1-step ungestured command	Uses spoon and cup
18 mo	Runs; throws objects from standing position	Turns pages 2-3 at a time; scribbles spontane-ously; builds tower of 3 blocks	7-10 word vocabulary; mature jargoning; knows body parts	Imitates parents in tasks/ chores; plays with other children

24 mo	Walks up and down stairs marking time	Imitates stroke with pencil; builds tower of 7 blocks; removes clothes	2-word sentences; ~ 50 word vocabulary; follows 2-step commands; uses pronouns (I, you, me) inappropriately	Parallel play
3 yr	Walks up stairs alternating feet; pedals tricycle	Copies a circle; undresses completely; dresses partially	3-word sentences; ≥ 250 word vocabulary; repeats 2 digits; uses pronouns correctly	Group play; shares toys; takes turns; knows name
4 yr	Alternates feet when descending stairs; hops; balances on 1 foot for ~5 sec	Copies a square; dresses completely; buttons clothes; catches ball	Says song/poem from memory; knows colors; asks questions	Tells "tall tales"; exaggerates
5 yr	Skips; jumps	Copies triangle; ties shoes	Prints name; follows 3-step commands; vocabulary too numerous to count	Abides by rules; competitive in play; helps with chores

Red Flags: Fisted hands beyond 3 months of age, persistence of primitive reflexes (moro reflex, asymmetric tonic neck reflex, or galant reflex, for example) beyond 6 months of age, and mouthing of objects beyond 9 months of age.

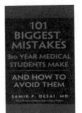

101 Biggest Mistakes 3rd Year Medical Students Make and How to Avoid Them

ISBN # 0-9725561-0-9

Compiled from discussions with hundreds of attending physicians, residents, and students, the *101 Biggest Mistakes 3rd Year Medical Students Make And How To Avoid Them* discusses the major mistakes that students make during this very important year. Avoiding these pitfalls is the key to third year success. This book will empower you, placing you in a position to have a successful experience, no matter what rotation or clerkship you are on. Once you are aware of these mistakes, you can do everything in your power to avoid them, thereby becoming the savvy student that is poised for clerkship success. Read what others have had to say:

"As someone who just matched into dermatology, I can tell you that residency program directors look closely at clerkship grades, especially for the more competitive residencies. *101 Biggest Mistakes 3rd Year Medical Students Make And How To Avoid Them* is a book that will help you get great clerkship grades."

—Review posted by Yang Xia on www.amazon.com

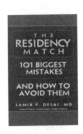

The Residency Match: 101 Biggest Mistakes And How To Avoid Them

ISBN # 0-9725561-1-7

Are there any steps you can take to maximize your chances of matching with the residency program of your choice? One of the keys is to become familiar with the major mistakes that students make during the residency application process. These are mistakes that are well known to residency program directors but are not familiar to many applicants. In *The Residency Match: 101 Biggest Mistakes And How To Avoid Them*, we not only show you these mistakes but also help you avoid them, placing you in a position for match success. Read what others have had to say:

"The fourth year of medical school can be a stressful, demanding time. This book cuts down on the amount of necessary reading that you must do in order to match well. It has tips about subjects I had not thought about (for example, you should have a case ready to present to your interviewer), as well as questions you will be asked in interviews and questions you should ask the interviewer. Overall, this is an easy-to-read book that I would definitely recommend because it contains all the essentials to matching in your ideal residency spot."

—Review posted by Jonathan Welch on www.amazon.com

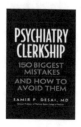

Psychiatry Clerkship: 150 Biggest Mistakes And How To Avoid Them

ISBN # 0-9725561-5-X

Many medical students find the psychiatry clerkship formidable, not because of a lack of knowledge about psychiatry, but because of a lack of preparation for actually doing the rotation.

This "insider's guide" can help you shave weeks off the learning curve by identifying the most common and deleterious mistakes that medical students make, as well as the best approaches to avoiding them. Plus, the "must know" information contained in the appendices will be an invaluable resource in answering questions during rounds and preparing for your exam.

"A student who reads this prior to starting the psychiatry clerkship will be primed for an excellent experience."

—Timothy K. Wolff, M.D., Psychiatry Clerkship Coordinator
Associate Professor of Psychiatry
University of Texas Southwestern Medical School

"This is a very useful and straightforward book that will successfully guide medical students through not only the psychiatry rotation, but many other clerkships as well."

—Anita Afzali, third year medical student
University of Washington School of Medicine

"The authors provide an astonishing amount of practical wisdom in easily understandable and readable prose. It deserves a place alongside the Washington manual in the pocket of every white coat in the halls of every medical school."

—Glenn O. Gabbard, M.D., Brown Foundation Chair of Psychoanalysis
Professor of Psychiatry
Baylor College of Medicine

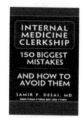

Internal Medicine Clerkship: 150 Biggest Mistakes And How To Avoid Them

ISBN # 0-9725561-2-5

Did you know that most medical students begin doing their best work at the end of the Internal Medicine clerkship? Wouldn't it be great if there were a book available that could speed up the learning curve so that students were performing at a high level right from the get-go? Now with the *Internal Medicine Clerkship: 150 Biggest Mistakes And How To Avoid Them*, there's absolutely no reason to save your best for last. Read what others have had to say:

"I read the book cover to cover prior to starting the rotation, and it helped me get off to a great start. I feel the book had a great influence on both my performance as a clinical student and my evaluation by my teammates. Overall, an extremely helpful and eye opening text. I attribute much of my success to the wisdom I gathered from this book."

—Brian Broaddus, after completing his Internal Medicine clerkship
at the Baylor College of Medicine

Surgery Clerkship: 150 Biggest Mistakes And How To Avoid Them
ISBN # 0-9725561-3-3

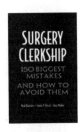

At most medical schools, the surgery clerkship is considered to be the most difficult rotation. Days start early, end late, and, from start to finish, the work is intense and demanding, often leading to physical and mental exhaustion. Of course, this can negatively impact your learning, enjoyment, and performance during the clerkship. To prevent this from happening, turn to the *Surgery Clerkship: 150 Biggest Mistakes and How To Avoid Them*, a resource that will help you overcome the challenges that await you. Lessen your anxiety, alleviate your fears, and position yourself for success by turning to the only book that will help you with every facet of the rotation, including not only your day to day patient care responsibilities but also your preparation for the oral and NBME clerkship exams.

"This new book will not only prepare the student for the tasks and responsibilities of surgical clerkship, but will provide a head start that is sure to impress."

—F. Charles Brunicardi, M.D., F.A.C.S.
DeBakey/Bard Professor
Chairman, Michael E. DeBakey Department of Surgery
Baylor College of Medicine

MD2B Titles

101 Biggest Mistakes 3rd Year Medical Students Make And How To Avoid Them

The Residency Match: 101 Biggest Mistakes And How To Avoid Them

Internal Medicine Clerkship: 150 Biggest Mistakes And How To Avoid Them

Surgery Clerkship: 150 Biggest Mistakes And How To Avoid Them

Pediatrics Clerkship: 101 Biggest Mistakes And How To Avoid Them

Psychiatry Clerkship: 150 Biggest Mistakes And How To Avoid Them

View sample chapters of these books at www.md2b.net

About www.md2b.net

Our website, www.md2b.net, is committed to helping today's medical student become tomorrow's doctor. The site is dedicated to providing students with the tools needed to tackle the challenges of medical school. The website provides the following information:

Survival Guides for 3rd Year Clerkships

Success tips (tips of the week)

Introduction to the residency match

Residency Match tips

—AND MUCH MORE!